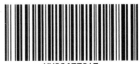

DO I HAVE DEMENTIA?

A REALISTIC GUIDE FOR WORRIERS

Dr. Joshua Johnson

ALSO BY JOSHUA L. JOHNSON

By the Fire in the House on the Hill

West Walk: Independence

DO I HAVE DEMENTIA?

A REALISTIC GUIDE FOR WORRIERS

DR. JOSHUA JOHNSON

First Printing, 2022
ISBN 978-1-7358849-2-9

Book cover design by Iskon Book Design
Book interior design by Iskon Book Design
Author photo by Jefferson Shallenberger

Cover drawing of a human cortical neuron by Santiago Ramon y Cajal. Reproduced courtesy of the Cajal Institute, Cajal Legacy, Spanish National Research Council (CSIC), Madrid, Spain.

With thanks to this book's first readers
and their marvelous middle-aged minds:
Colleen, Tim, Noah, and Jennifer.

CONTENTS

INTRODUCTION

I felt a Cleaving in my Mind—
As if my Brain had split—
I tried to match it—Seam by Seam—
But could not make them fit.

The thought behind, I strove to join
Unto the thought before—
But Sequence ravelled out of reach
Like Balls—upon a Floor.

EMILY DICKINSON

I have worried, since age 20, that I am developing dementia.

Most of us worry about ourselves. We worry about our health. We notice a symptom—a muscle twitch, change in vision, new headache, palpitation—and worry that something has changed in our bodies for the worse. We worry that something is wrong with us. Perhaps body worry begins in adolescence, when many of us compare our appearances with others and find the shortfalls;

and then, as we age, the scope of self-awareness is widened to encompass not just the body's flawed appearance but its fallibility. The new car becomes the old car, and we drive, listening closely for ominous noises of dysfunction. The body, like a modern car, comes with many sensors that apprise us of its status and immediate environment: temperature, pressure, pain, limb position, ambient light and sound and smell; fuel and fluid status; even the waste is monitored. The information is useful, even critical. Yet it is possible that the body gives us more information than we need. Human sensory input is routed through a processor more complex, self-conscious, and idiosyncratic than any car's computer: the human brain. Simple sensory data enter the mind, where, under the influence of self-consciousness and emotion, a symptom is produced.

My symptom—my worry for incipient dementia—has been present my entire adult life, thus demonstrating its folly. I do not remember the specifics of my state of mind as a young adult, but I recall being a freshman in college and spending a day in the medical library researching early-onset Alzheimer's disease. I seriously thought this could be my diagnosis. I was twenty years old, and my coursework included calculus, chemistry, and a new language's steep learning curve. That I could succeed in school yet be sincerely concerned about mental decline is laughable now but perhaps not unique; Emily Dickinson, in the poem quoted above, similarly sees her mind—keen, creative, quick, young—as disintegrating. The irrational worry for dementia illuminates the psychopathology of the impulse: we worry despite reliable evidence that worry is unnecessary. That same, durable psychopathology eventually found an end route in my mind: the older I get the more I wonder if my college worry was in fact a presentiment of my appointment in Samarra not with death but with dementia.

After my visit to the library in college I concluded that I did not have early Alzheimer's. In fact, I simply had an imperfect human mind. As a physician I see the difficulty that young people have in accommodating to their first serious health problem: they do not yet understand that their bodies are imperfect and can fail.

Although I was cognitively normal as a college freshman, the specter of dementia has followed me. Sometimes, when my mind is working well and I have made no more boneheaded errors than can be expected for a imperfect person in an imperfect world, the specter is as distant as I imagine it must be for those people gifted with powerful memories whom I envy when they say, with offhanded confidence, something like, "No, it's ok. I don't need to write it down. I'll remember." Other times—in a conversation in which I forget an actor's name, when I walk into the kitchen and immediately forget my purpose, when I quickly forget an acquaintance's name, when I forget how to spell "acquaintance"— dementia lays its hand on my shoulder and freshens the worry.

I know that I am not the only person concerned for their memory. Emily Dickinson expresses this same concern: a sense of losing grasp of thoughts, of a fragmented, dysfunctional, "ravelling" mind. In my work as a neurologist I regularly see patients with this complaint. Those patients under age 65 are usually neurologically well. Their brain is normal and disease-free but is overwhelmed by fixable problems: poor sleep, mood issues, chronic pain, medication side-effects, or just an overly stressful life. Others, particularly older patients, are more likely to have a disease such as Alzheimer's. Many of us look to these older people—hunched over walkers, eyes dim, wrangling their spent bodies and minds to complete even simple tasks—and see our future selves. The worry is always fresh.

Having seen many neurologically normal patients concerned for their cognitive function, I wished to share with a larger audience and in greater depth the path through this very particular worry: that one is losing one's mind.

The path begins with an understanding of normal. What is normal aging for a human brain? As most of us age our cognitive power diminishes to the same degree as the function of our other organs. Our skin loses elasticity, our eyes require correction, our hair thins, our muscles lose strength and speed, our hearts do not support the same level of exertion as when we were twenty. Similarly, by the fifth or six decade, our minds do not work as quickly or as surely as they once did. Names are more easily forgotten. Simple math requires greater concentration. Details of yesterday's conversation vanish. This is normal aging. We cannot expect better than this. It is the natural history of central nervous system neurons to mature and then faithfully power the mind for decades before the connections fizzle, conduction slows, and cells die, such that the name of your neighbor's second child comes easily to mind one day and is nowhere to be found the next. There are rare individuals—the cognitive supermodels for their age, admired and resented, outstanding and bizarre—whose cognitive power does not decline, and at age 85 they are as quick in a conversation as in middle age. We must not dwell on these individuals; they are aberrations. Their gift cannot be shared, and we cannot expect to be like them. We—the normal people—have a different path to follow in our cognitive journey, and we must keep our heads down, adjust expectations, and pretend not to notice when the ancient cognitive supermodels speak, without searching for words, about their cruise on the Volga two years past, naming each town sequentially and with a proper Russian accent. Flaunting it. To compare oneself with them only hones worry to a finer edge.

So what can normal people expect of their memory as they age? The normal arc of memory function is a long one. While on the arc, worry may make one feel as if the downward drop is about to accelerate, that the smooth, shallow curve will soon bend precipitously. Many people concerned for their memory look back at their cognitive power earlier in life and overestimate it, believing that their memory was once much better than it actually was. My library visit in college has been a useful signpost for me in my concern for dementia, for it tells me that there was never really a time when my memory was exceptional. I have come to see this diminishing arc of cognitive power as reassuring, in a way, because it is expected. The normal arc of cognitive power moves slowly downwards over many decades. It is normal to forget. The key question is: When is the forgetting greater than expected for age?

I was tempted to subtitle this book *A Worrier's Guide* but decided against it because such a title would imply that the book's aim is to reassure, to convince the reader that everything will be fine, that the risk for dementia is negligible, and that there is no need for worry. Such a book could also be subtitled *A Guide to Assuage the Worried* and it would de-emphasize or even hide risk. It would examine cognitive aging exclusively from an optimistic perspective. It would not challenge readers to develop an accurate understanding of the complexities of cognitive aging. Although the book would temporarily dispel worry, it could not be a solution to worry. A book that selects data for the sake of reassurance would give readers a very poor understanding of the true nature of cognitive aging. And when cognitive mis-firings recurred, as they inevitably would, readers would find themselves ill equipped to comprehend the problem.

In fact, a scientifically and emotionally honest book cannot be written in which the specter of dementia is routed. Confronting the possibility of dementia is to confront very hard truths. It can be like confronting the possibility of death; both mark the end of a life and the letting go of the self. There is nothing easy about this. To look at these truths about dementia squarely requires fortitude, an open mind, and a willingness to accept that even in the absence of dementia our competencies, over a lifespan, do not remain the same. Books that claim to cure dementia or that make assurances that dementia is entirely preventable are beguiling because they confirm what we wish to be true. But such books defraud their readers. They are dishonest in their representation of the facts about dementia, or they ignore established facts, confecting opinions by selecting only data that rationalizes their claims. To inaccurately understate the real possibility of dementia, to make claims for interventions that will certainly prevent it, to say that Alzheimer's disease is curable, is to lie.

This book promises to be honest with the reader. Some facts will be difficult to read, and there will be moments of deflation when we confront hard realities, for example, when in chapter 7 we examine dementia risk in the context of a family history of Alzheimer's disease. These moments are inevitable, I think, in a book that truthfully discusses the facts of cognitive life. But there will be other moments—and I hope that finishing the book provides a lasting moment of this kind—when the value of a clear understanding of dementia risk prevails over worry or at least diminishes it, limits it, and confines it to a smaller and more manageable territory within our imaginations. Many readers will finish chapter 7 feeling not deflated but reassured that their actual risk for dementia is less than they previously believed.

Overall, this book tries to represent the dilemma of cognitive aging (*Are my cognitive symptoms normal for age, or do I have dementia?*) realistically, as a good physician might present it to a patient: frankly, evenhandedly acknowledging both the presence of risk and the (much greater) possibility of dementia-free aging, supporting conclusions with fact, and using only reliable data as a basis for recommendations. (Please see footnote[1] regarding the data used in this book.) I hope that readers also discover some very positive aspects of aging that counterbalance those facts more difficult to hear. My wish is to leave readers with a clear,

---

[1] For the purposes of this book, "reliable data" or "good data" ideally means data supported by more than a single prospective trial of large numbers of participants, randomized and controlled when possible, and peer-reviewed and edited. This book does not consider quality data to include studies of small numbers of participants, anecdotal studies, studies of non-humans, *in vitro* studies, small imaging series, or studies with counterintuitive and novel conclusions that are unsupported by previous research or not reproduced in subsequent studies. When suboptimal data is used in this book it is acknowledged and conclusions hedged.

realistic sense of the facts of cognitive life, whether favorable or unfavorable, thus robbing worry of one of its chief levers—ignorance—and enhancing readers' sense of their own competence in knowing when forgetfulness is normal for age, or when it isn't.

When is forgetting greater than expected for age? This is, of course, the question that lurks. The question is answerable, even if we dread the answer. Perhaps we even think that raising the question at all implies the affirmative: we would not question our cognitive health if something were not amiss. The available non-academic literature—found in the bookstore under the genres "Health," "Medical," or "Self-Help"—is focused on the experience of the patient, family, or caregiver once the diagnosis of dementia is made, yet there is no good resource for the person who wonders if their mind's decline is greater than should be expected for age. This book is for that person. In it, we will discuss normal cognitive function over a lifespan. We will identify problems that can look like dementia but are not. We will define what dementia is, and we will discuss factors that may increase the risk of acquiring it. We will consider perhaps the most powerful provoker of worry—a family history of dementia—and examine in detail the genetic elements that influence the likelihood of developing Alzheimer's disease. And we will briefly examine some simple, data-based ideas for preserving cognitive health.

Having mapped the many factors that influence the likelihood that you, the reader, will develop dementia, the book's final chapter questions the premise that dementia is to be dreaded. Can we be certain that life with dementia is poor? Dementia induces confusion, radical changes in competence, and loss of lifelong cognitive pleasures. Yet might there be some benefit in downsizing the mind? I am not making light; I am looking—as this book seeks to do for the reader—for a portal of positivity in a fearful diagnosis. Our world exists only in our minds; therefore, provided all basic needs are met, might the closer quarters of the demented mind be cozy? Could dementia be a pleasurable kind of myopia, as in drunkenness but different, the sensorium ice water clear? Is the demented person staring out the window in fact seeing the world in a way that others cannot, with a perception more simple, essential, clear, and vivid? The demented state is sometimes called "a second childhood", but perhaps instead of fearing it we may experience it as we did our first childhood: life radically new, intimidating, and beyond our control. Don't all worthwhile things start this way?

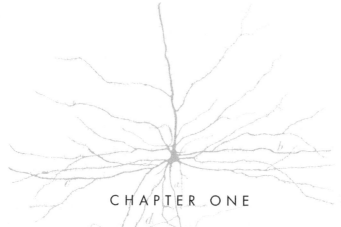

CHAPTER ONE

WHAT IS DEMENTIA?

I was called "demented" as a kid. At the time I didn't take it seriously because it was a common put-down, and I called other kids "demented", too. Being called "demented" in elementary school meant that you were mentally abnormal, perverse, maybe crazy, dim though not totally witless. Its meaning was similar to, but a little bit sharper than, the original meaning of the word "queer:" crooked where others were straight; twisted. Marty Feldman's character, Igor, in the movie *Young Frankenstein*, captures the meaning of "demented" both in his appearance—skeleton-white face, crooked nose, bulging walleyes—and behavior, as when he chooses an abnormal specimen for a brain transplant, reading its label as "Abby Normal." In the same wacky vein, a Bay Area DJ with a weekend radio program when I was in high school called himself "Dr. Demento." His schtick was to talk in a kooky, high voice—like Rick Steves on helium—and play off-color records à la Weird Al Yankovic. Query "dementia" in a thesaurus and the following words are listed as synonyms: mental disorder, derangement, insanity, madness, unbalanced. The implication is that "dementia" is an emotional or psychiatric problem.

Yet this usage is in contrast with the word as used by current medical science—yet another example of perfectly good medical nomenclature corrupted by general usage. These days, such words as "dumb", "retarded", "mental", "cripple"—and "walleyed"—make us cringe, as they should, but it is worth noting that these words once had a specific, descriptive objectivity quite apart from their later stigmatizing use by the public. Even so, the use of the term "dementia" has somehow clung to is medical roots, thesauruses and children notwithstanding, perhaps because there is no good alternative term available. Dementia, as the term is used by modern medical science, is a condition of progressive cognitive decline that is abnormal for age, caused by a disease in the brain itself, and results in impairment of memory, mental processing, or judgement.

"Dementia" is a general term. Saying that someone has "dementia" is as nonspecific as saying that someone has "an infection;" a better understanding requires further specification, such as "lung infection" or "skin infection". Within the general category of "dementia" are specific dementias, each with its own name and characteristics.

The most common dementias (accounting for 95% of all dementias) are Alzheimer's disease, vascular dementia, dementia with Lewy Bodies, Parkinson's dementia, Frontotemporal dementia, and Normal Pressure Hydrocephalus.[1] (These are the dementias that will be discussed in chapter 6.) Each dementia has its own name because each has distinct features considered typical of that disease. Dementia with Lewy Bodies, for example, is named for the appearance under the microscope of the brains of people suffering

---

[1] Gupta S, et al. Rare and Unusual Dementias. *Advances in psychiatric treatment* 2009;15: 364–371 DOI: 10.1192/apt.bp.107.003558

from the disease ("Lewy bodies" are seen within the brain cells), as well as for the symptoms typical of the disease such as forgetfulness, hallucinations, and movement abnormalities. While each dementia has features that are considered typical, there is actually a good deal of overlap between them, such that dementia with Lewy bodies can look a lot like the dementia of Parkinson's disease (they both cause problems with walking and other movements), and the behavioral problems that sometimes occur in Alzheimer's disease can resemble those in frontotemporal dementia. Sometimes this overlap makes it difficult to know exactly which dementia a person has, but usually, as the dementia progresses over months to years, the diagnosis becomes clear.

It is important to clarify what dementia is not. Schizophrenia, bipolar disorder, depression, compulsions, or anxiety are not dementia. (In contrast to the thesaurus' suggestions, dementia is not the same as craziness or insanity.) The cognitive side effects of medications or drugs are not dementia. One is not demented if suffering from delirium, which is a temporary confusion caused by another medical condition such as organ dysfunction or an infection. These conditions are either psychiatric, non-progressive, or are caused mainly by problems with organs besides the brain. Dementia, in contrast, is a condition of progressive cognitive decline that is abnormal for age, progressive, and caused by a disease in the brain itself.[2]

In beginning this book with a definition of dementia I do not mean to stoke fears—though this might be a good technique for

---

[2] Some published papers also include among the dementias brain injuries such as cerebral palsy or brain trauma, but these conditions are not relevant to the topic of new memory concerns in the aging and are not included in our discussion.

compelling readers to continue reading. In fact, misunderstandings about the nature of dementia are common. Having read this short chapter, for instance, some people will realize that their concern for a genetic dementia was based on a mistake: a mother with bipolar disorder is, in fact, not the same thing as a mother with dementia. We begin with a definition of dementia in order to build an understanding of cognition and aging from the ground up. The first level—this chapter—clarifies the terms of worry: what, exactly, dementia is. The next level—chapter two—builds on our understanding by showing what cognitive aging looks like in people without dementia. It is my hope that each chapter adds to the understanding acquired in the previous chapter, with the ultimate goal of a firm grasp of the cognitive facts of life: what normal cognition is, the line between normal and abnormal cognition, and the elements of dementia risk.

🔔 REMEMBER:

✓ "Dementia" is a general category, within which are dementias with specific names.

✓ Dementia is a condition of progressive cognitive decline that is abnormal for age and results in impairment of memory, mental processing, or judgement.

✓ Dementia is *not*: schizophrenia, bipolar disorder, depression, compulsions, anxiety, drug or
medication side effects, or the cognitive effects of
dysfunction of other organs such as the thyroid,
kidneys, liver, or heart.

✓ 95% of all dementia cases are due to Alzheimer's
dementia, vascular dementia, dementia with Lewy
bodies, Parkinson's dementia, frontotemporal dementia, or normal pressure hydrocephalus. The
specific features of these dementias are discussed
in chapter 6.

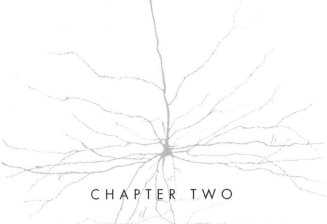

CHAPTER TWO

WHAT IS NORMAL BRAIN AGING?

The parents at the school auction sip wine, cup hors d'oeuvre in little napkins, converse politely, and stroll among the auction items with the patient curiosity of well-to-do museum goers. Indeed, they are more than parents. They are society's crucial middle-aged workers: the fixers, producers, managers, and planners. They are important members of the team of adults that keeps the gears of civilization in good order. They are the grownups. As middle-aged adults, they have more resources—material and cognitive—than any other age group. And the world's good order depends, to some extent, on each of them. You, too, are a parent and team member—yet when you realize this, you begin doubt the integrity of the system.

"Wait a minute," you balk. "We are in charge?"

For you have recently begun to wonder whether you are indeed a dependable member of the grownup team. Lately, you have noticed a change in your brain's behavior. Your mind sometimes betrays you. Names do not come as quickly and reliably as when you were younger. You walk into a room

and forget why you're there. You make small mistakes with
numbers. You forget the plot of the TV series you watched
a couple weeks ago. On the other hand, your career has not
suffered, and you have confidence in your work. In fact, you're
better than ever at your job. Should you worry?

► Cognitive mistakes are not necessarily the warning signs of dementia. The brain ages, and cognitive power declines. This can be normal for age.

► Some brain anatomy and cognitive skills mature in adolescence.

► Other parts of the brain mature in mid-life and are important in cognitive tasks involving practiced skills, judgment, problem solving, and wisdom.

► All cognitive abilities begin to decline in middle age.

► A certain amount of forgetfulness and mental slowness is a normal and expected part of cognitive aging.

► *Read on to learn more.*

PART 1: THE ADOLESCENT BRAIN

Brains change. There is no finish line for brain development, no moment of completion that is as easily identified as height, shoe size, or lung capacity. The brain development of infants and children is spectacular, but less obvious brain growth continues well into our fifth decade—even as the rest of the body is in decline. Change defines the brain at all ages.

Our expectations for our own minds must therefore also change as we age. The middle-aged mind is probably the most powerful of all minds, yet it is in middle age that a change in the cognitive terrain first becomes perceptible: the mind's pace slows, its footing becomes less sure, and each stride—each cognitive task—requires a little more effort.

Memory and thinking speed diminish with age. Is this really normal? Work and pleasure rely on certain cognitive abilities, and impairment would be life changing. When is change abnormal? When does it indicate a disease? How to know?

The first question (*Can cognitive change be normal?*) is examined in this chapter, while the subsequent question (*When are cognitive symptoms abnormal?*) is addressed later in the book. Worry for dementia may urge you to skip this chapter and proceed directly to later chapters, but reconsider: this chapter will briefly examine the fundamentals of normal cognitive aging from adolescence to old age, providing a background for understanding worrisome cognitive symptoms.

The story of the aging brain begins at an important developmental moment: adolescence. The shape and size of a child's brain are similar to an adult's (by two years of age the brain has reached

80% of its adult size) but it is still undergoing important changes. To understand these changes we must grasp a few basic facts about the brain: we need to know about neurons, axons, and myelin.

Neurons are very specialized cells that are found only in the brain, spinal cord, and nerves. The basic parts of a neuron are the cell body, which contains DNA and other machinery for basic cell maintenance, and the axon, which is a long extension from the cell body that connects with other neurons via the axon terminal.

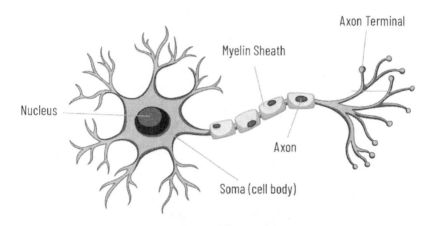

Figure 1: Anatomy of a neuron

The purpose of neurons is to communicate with other cells. If, for example, you to wish to shake someone's hand, neurons in the brain send electrical signals down their axons[1] to other neurons in the spinal cord, triggering in turn a signal in spinal cord neurons that conducts down their axons and into the nerves in the arm, then to the hand, which then lifts, extends, and makes the handshake. Everything we do is dependent on the function

---

[1] Axons can be short or up to several feet long.

of neurons and axons: moving, feeling, seeing, smelling, thinking. Fundamentally, thinking (reading this sentence) and remembering are just this: the coordinated activity of millions of neurons, their axons, and the signaling between them.

Signaling by axons is aided by myelin, which increases the speed and efficiency of signal conduction along the axon. Myelin is a substance that is wrapped in layers around the axon like a seashell's spirals around a center. The following image displays an axon that has been cut in two with the end turned toward the viewer.

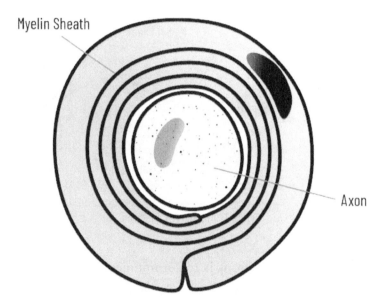

Figure 2: Myelin around an axon

Now, a little more anatomy to help us understand the cognitive changes of early and middle life. The brain's outer rim, or "cortex" (also called "gray matter") contains many neurons. The thickness of the cortex is determined by the number of neurons and their connections. From the cortex, neurons extend their axons (which are surrounded by myelin) deep into the brain's "white matter" (which takes its coloration from the myelin itself).[2]

In adolescence, neurons[3] are still undergoing important changes. Axons grow and increase their connections to other neurons. Myelin thickens and matures around the axons. These changes proceed in a predictable, organized pattern—for instance, myelin matures first at the back of the brain, then progresses forward, with the front of the brain's myelin maturing last.

With late adolescence, however, the trajectory of brain development radically shifts. Its development to this point makes sense: neurons must mature—lengthening their axons, growing myelin, increasing the number of connections between neurons—to enable their special function of signaling between cells. But in late adolescence, development makes a counterintuitive break. The adolescent brain simplifies itself. Synaptic connections are cropped, axonal complexity reduced, and the robust brain growth so diligently cultivated since conception is overhauled. Not all of childhood's brain survives into adulthood; in the transition to maturity, brain is shed. One researcher of the anatomy of cognitive aging explains the events of adolescence:[4]

> Gray matter loss during this period reflects a sculpting process of the
> immature brain into the fully functioning mature one…Connections

---

[2] White matter and gray matter are named after the appearance of these tissues in cadavers.

[3] This book's cover features an illustration of a human cortical neuron drawn by the 19th century neuroscientist and Nobel laureate Santiago Ramón y Cajal.

[4] Casey BJ, et al. Imaging the developing brain: what have we learned about cognitive development? *TRENDS in Cognitive Sciences* 2005;9(3)

are being fine-tuned with the elimination of an overabundance of synapses and strengthening of relevant connections with development and experience.

There is purpose in this process of brain simplification. The brain emerges from adolescence as if purged. It is lean, trim, quick, fluid, and incisive. It is an organ fit for survival. The remaining connections between neurons are strengthened, the gray matter density is maximized, and myelin is growing.

Now we can start to see how these changes in brain maturity are reflected in cognition itself. In some ways, the post-adolescent brain is on a lifetime high. It is quick and flexible, able to engage in multiple tasks at once and shift between them easily. It can quickly learn new information, problem-solve, and identify and remember complex patterns. These cognitive abilities are elements of "fluid intelligence". Fluid intelligence is the raw processing power of the brain. It is characterized as "abilities involving problem-solving and reasoning about things that are less familiar and are independent of what one has learned. Fluid cognition includes a person's innate ability to process and learn new information, solve problems, and attend to and manipulate one's environment."[5] The young dominate the older in games that exploit fluid intelligence and require quick recall, rapid information synthesize, and quick changes of plan. They are better at memorizing the placement of playing cards, for example, or rapid-recall games such as *Catchphrase* (in which a movie, book, famous person, or

---

[5] Harada CN, et al. Normal Cognitive Aging. *Clin Geriatr Med* 2013;29(4):737–752. DOI:10.1016/j.cger.2013.07.002

event must be quickly named), or following the serial addition of a Blackjack game without error.

Fluid intelligence peaks very early in life, at about age 20. We aren't aware of this peak, because when it happens we are barely out of adolescence and, despite our powerful brains, we are kind of clueless. At age 20, our fluid intelligence is peaking—and it then declines linearly for the rest of our lives. The following graph illustrates this decline by plotting the components of fluid intelligence (working memory, short term memory, speed of processing) over time.[6]

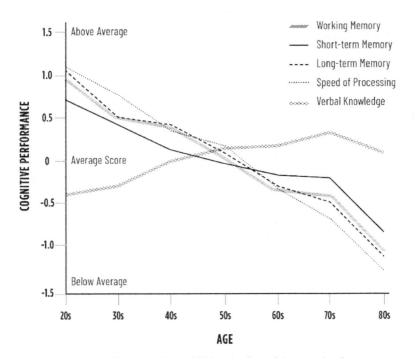

Figure 3: Most cognitive abilities decline with normal aging
(Adapted from: Park DC, et al. Models of Visuospatial and Verbal Memory Across the Adult Life Span. Psychology and Aging 2002;17 (2): 299–320.)

---

6 Park DC, et al. Models of Visuospatial and Verbal Memory Across the Adult Life Span. *Psychology and Aging* 2002;17 (2): 299–320.. DOI: 10.1037//0882-7974.17.2.299

On this graph's vertical axis, an average cognitive score is 0. People ages 20-40 score above average in most domains, including short-term memory, long-term memory, speed of cognitive processing, and working memory.[7] We see that 20-year-olds perform best in these tasks. With every decade after age 20 there is a regular decline in fluid intelligence, falling below average by about age 50.

Fluid intelligence declines with age. How does this manifest in real life? Though the graph, above, demonstrates a decline in fluid intelligence beginning at age 20, most people do not actually notice a significant change until about age 40, when certain small cognitive tasks require more effort and concentration. In middle age it becomes more difficult to hold several numbers in the mind at once; for instance, it is an effort to remember a check number, check date, and check amount all at the same time. Even simple math requires more concentration. New task learning and problem-solving are slower.

Fortunately, there is more to the story of cognitive aging than a decline in fluid intelligence. Earlier, this chapter stated that the middle-aged mind is "probably the most powerful of all minds." How can this be, if a twenty-year-old mind's fluid intelligence is so obviously superior to a 50-year-old's? The answer is that there is more to human intelligence than fluid intelligence. Re-examine the graph of memory and processing speed shown earlier. In contrast to the regular decline of fluid intelligence, one component of intelligence does not diminish. Verbal knowledge follows a different course: it increases with age.

---

[7] "Working memory" processes, stores, and maintains visual or auditory information for short-term use.

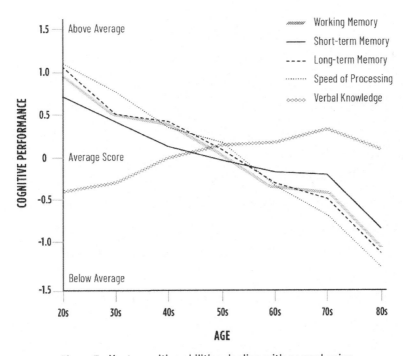

Figure 3: Most cognitive abilities decline with normal aging

(Adapted from: Park DC, et al. Models of Visuospatial and Verbal Memory Across the Adult Life Span. Psychology and Aging 2002;17 (2): 299-320.)

Verbal knowledge—the understanding and use of language—is a component of "crystalized intelligence." Crystalized intelligence, in turn, is "skills, ability, and knowledge that is over-learned, well-practiced, and familiar,"[8] and "depends on learning and cultural influences and reflects experience, breadth of knowledge, comprehension, judgment, and wisdom."[9] It is the kind of

---

[8] Aine CJ, et al. Development and Decline of Memory Functions in Normal, Pathological and Healthy Successful Aging. *Brain Topogr* 2011; 24(3-4): 323–339. DOI:10.1007/s10548-011-0178-x

[9] Craik FIM, Bialystok E. Cognition through the lifespan: mechanisms of change. *TRENDS in Cognitive Sciences* 2006;10(3). DOI: 10.1016/j.tics.2006.01.007

intelligence that is strengthened over a lifetime, the value-added of life experience, which is why, in the graph above, verbal knowledge is below average in 20-year-olds. General intelligence—what we mean when we say someone is "smart"—is a combination of fluid intelligence and crystalized intelligence; the two components are complementary. Fluid intelligence is a 90 WPM keyboardist taking dictation while simultaneously editing its content, while crystalized intelligence is the novelist or journalist carefully dictating a work of complexity involving an acquired knowledge of culture, language, history, politics, or psychology.

Although fluid intelligence declines after age 20, in middle age there is stability of cognitive power because crystallized intelligence is still growing. While there may be a noticeable decline in the fluid aspect of general intelligence, there is still a sustained ability to do effective cognitive work (as proven by your success in following the meaning of this information-dense chapter). The reason that middle-aged (and older) brains can still do effective work is the brain's increasing inclination to apply crystalized intelligence in problem-solving.

The tendency to rely on crystalized intelligence has an anatomical basis that is explored in the second part of this chapter. But first let's consider the cases of two people, Carol and her mother, Millie (both names have been changed). Carol is middle-aged, and her aging mother's forgetfulness makes Carol wonder about her own memory.

Carol and Millie: The forgetting list

Carol secretly understands her mother. Millie is almost 80, and she forgets things. Carol watches her mother and doesn't think that her forgetfulness is different than other older people's. Once a week, Millie's friends meet for happy hour at Carol's house. They play poker and drink Old Fashioneds, and Carol overhears stories about the things they have forgotten. These stories are different than their complaints about their knees or their bowels—complaints with a mildly tragic, woe-is-me quality intended to earn sympathy, which they savor for a while before someone else mentions bladder trouble, or back pain, followed by clucks of support all around until eventually the sympathy is as fairly dealt among them as the playing cards.

But the talk about forgetfulness is different. These aged ladies treat forgetting as funny. In preparation for happy hour, they write down the things they have forgotten that week. All week, they carry around a pencil and a list—like a shopping list but meant to record the things they have forgotten. Carol doesn't know how it started, but now the "forgetting list" is the ladies' second favorite part of happy hour, after the Old Fashioneds. Right about the time the maraschino cherries begin to appear among the ice at the bottom of their glasses, someone takes out her list. Then the cards are put aside and Carol, in the kitchen, hears their laughter. Carol thinks it is an unusual but probably healthy way to share the difficulties of being old. Carol admires the ladies' resourcefulness: they are literally making fun of their problems. Carol believes that it takes a kind wisdom to do that—and courage.

Carol understands her mother. She knows her preferences, she knows how she will react in most situations, she knows the kind of clothes she likes and her sizes, she knows her favorites among family and friends. But she also understands her mother in a secret way. Carol, too, knows what it is like to forget.

Her mother forgets regularly. She lives with Carol because someday—not now, but someday—she will need extra help, either because her memory will worsen or because she will have other health problems that will make it difficult to care for herself. Carol already does her mother's finances but otherwise Millie is independent, cooking several meals each week and doing everything else herself, including driving. But they both know that there may be a time when she cannot do these things.

Carol sympathizes—and not just as a daughter watching her mother age. Carol, too, makes mistakes. Her own memory is limited. She was shocked once to overhear on the happy hour "forgetting list" an error that she herself had made: she called her internet provider to upgrade her service, and between dialing and the representative's answer she forgot whom she was calling. (To be fair, she was doing several things at once and was distracted. And once the person answered it took Carol only a second or two to remember what she was doing.)

She doesn't want to understand her mother in this way. She isn't almost 80, like her mother; she's only 52.

The forgetfulness that Carol experiences is predictable and probably normal. Fluid intelligence declines from our twenties onward. The speed and agility of Carol's 52-year-old brain—its fluid intelligence—has declined since her 20s. She did not notice this when she was 30, but she notices it now. She is a financial advisor, and it has become clear to her that her mental power with numbers isn't what it was. At the same time, she knows that her understanding of the economy and investments is much broader, deeper, and more nuanced than when she started her work in her mid-20s. In other words, her intelligence is well-crystalized by learning and experience. How is it that, on one hand, her mind increasingly struggles with some tasks, while in some ways her brain seems to work better than ever?

PART 2: THE AGING BRAIN

To understand how some aspects of cognition—such as fluid intelligence—can be in decline while others—crystallized intelligence—thrive, we must understand more about neurons and myelin.

Recall that neurons' main function is to communicate with other cells. Myelin helps with this communication by increasing the speed of signal conduction along axons. But we are not born with our axons fully myelinated. Complete myelination of the brain takes decades. The following graph demonstrates the maturation of gray matter (containing neurons and their connections) and white matter (comprised of axons and their myelin).[10]

---

[10] Aine CJ, et al. Development and Decline of Memory Functions in Normal, Pathological and Healthy Successful Aging. *Brain Topogr* 2011; 24(3-4): 323–339. DOI:10.1007/s10548-011-0178-x

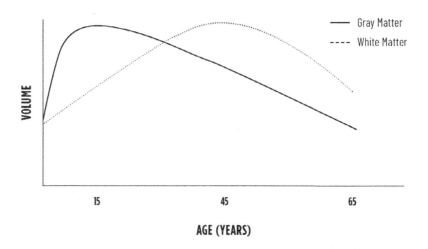

Figure 4: Changes in brain gray matter and white matter volumes

(Adapted from: Aine CJ, et al. Development and Decline of Memory Functions in Normal, Pathological and Healthy Successful Aging. Brain Topogr 2011; 24(3-4): 323-339.)

We see from this graph that the volume of gray matter (made of neurons in the cortex) is maximal by late adolescence. White matter (made of axons and myelin), on the other hand, follows a different path, peaking in middle age. These two facts—the maturation of gray matter when young, and the maturation of white matter in middle age—help explain why cognition changes with age. When young, the maturation of the cortex and the neurons within it establish the rote processing power of the brain, a person's "innate ability to process and learn new information, solve problems, and attend to and manipulate one's environment." These are the abilities that Carol enjoyed early in her career: effortless math, sharp short-term memory, quick learning, reliable multi-tasking. So, what about the other arc in the graph above, the one that shows that white matter matures later than gray matter? Does this influence cognitive aging?

The answer is yes. The relatively late maturation of the brain's white matter is the reason that the ability to do complex cognitive tasks reaches its apex in middle age. In particular, it is the late maturation of the white matter in a part of the brain called the "frontal lobes" that is most important in the timing of cognitive maturity.

Every brain has two frontal lobes. We see the left frontal lobe in this image of the brain as viewed from the left side.

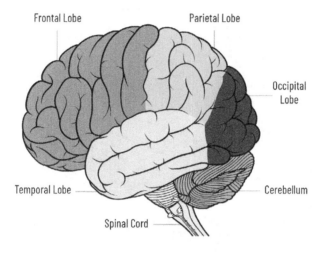

Figure 5: Human brain anatomy

The frontal lobes have several important functions, including motor control (strength) in the body. In terms of cognition, however, there is no more important part of the frontal lobes than the prefrontal cortex (PFC). The PFC is "the most versatile structure in the brain."[11] It has intellectual range, adaptability, and depth. It is the anatomical seat of human maturity, wisdom,

[11] Park DC, Reuter-Lorenz P. The Adaptive Brain: Aging and Neurocognitive Scaffolding. *Annu Rev Psychol* 2009;60: 173–196. DOI: 10.1146/annurev.psych.59.103006.093656

insight, and complex, associative thought. It governs "executive function", which entails the "capacities that allow a person to successfully engage in independent, appropriate, purposive, and self-serving behavior. This includes a wide range of cognitive abilities such as the ability to self-monitor, plan, organize, reason, be mentally flexible, and problem solve."[12]

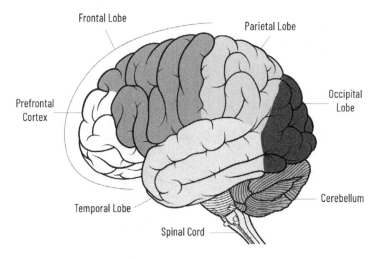

Figure 6: The prefrontal cortex

Without the frontal lobes' prefrontal cortex, we would begin tasks but not finish them. Planning would be disorganized and ineffective. Projects would be stalled by any unanticipated developments that required spontaneous problem solving and re-direction. Solutions would be reflexive and superficial, and they would overlook consequences. Without the PFC in charge, a task would be as messy, disorganized, and chaotic as an adolescent's bedroom.

[12] Harada CN, et al. Normal Cognitive Aging. *Clin Geriatr Med* 2013;29(4):737–752. DOI:10.1016/j.cger.2013.07.002

The PFC matures among the last of all brain structures. Its white matter is not fully myelinated until about age 50. No other organ has a similar developmental arc. By age 50, many people must wear glasses. Joints are more easily strained, physical labor is more difficult, hair thins, muscle mass diminishes, blood pressure and glucose levels rise, and, overall, the body begins to appear past its prime. Yet at the same time, the PFC is just reaching its maximal white matter volume. The timing of PFC maturity is why the middle-aged brain is the most powerful brain. It is the anatomical basis for crystallized intelligence. Youth may be speedier, but the middle-aged mind has cognitive depth and breadth, with emotional and intellectual maturity and a knowledge base that is fully crystalized by experience.

The prefrontal cortex matures last of all brain parts, and it is unfortunately also the first to show the effects of middle age. Researchers propose a "last in, first out" hypothesis for human brain development: those parts that mature last, such as the prefrontal cortex, are also the first to decline. This pattern is demonstrated by MRI, other imaging techniques, and post-mortem studies: by late middle age, the gray and white matter of the frontal lobes are in simultaneous decline.

But the prefrontal cortex adapts even in its decline. In young people, executive function is supported mainly by the left prefrontal cortex, with use of the right PFC only when tasks become very difficult and require much concentration. Older people, on the other hand, demonstrate a regular tendency to use both the right and left PFC. In this way, executive function sustains good working order even late in life, and cognitive strength persists for years despite the late-middle age decline in brain volume.

Eventually, however, the linear decline in gray matter (since age 20) and white matter (since age 50) manifest in a noticeable loss of cognitive power. The symptoms are familiar: forgetfulness, substantial word-finding trouble, misplaced keys, overall slowness (in the grocery store self-checkout line, ordering at a restaurant, learning a new cell phone app, processing moderately complex financial information), and a general inability to keep up with others in conversation and learning. One older writer describes memory's pitfalls in old age:[13]

> My conversation may be full of holes and pauses, but I've learned to dispatch a private Apache scout ahead into the next sentence, the one coming up, to see if there are any vacant names or verbs in the landscape up there. If he sends back a warning, I'll pause meaningfully, duh, until something else comes to mind.

Carol thinks she notices early signs of these memory troubles in herself. She can do math, though without the speed and confidence she once had. She cannot hold multiple numbers in her head, but she clearly understands their implications and relevance to the economy and her clients' investment plans. On Monday, she does not always remember where the NASDAQ finished on Friday, but she is clear in her understanding of the overall market, the movements of its sectors, the current interest rate, the Federal Reserve's position on the economy, and historical precedents for today's market. Because she is human, and aging, her brain is changing; but her brain still works very well.

---

[13] Roger Angell, *The New Yorker*, 2/9/14

It is important to emphasize that the changes in intelligence over a lifespan that are described in this chapter are predictable, which is to say that they are normal. It is perhaps surprising that our most effective tool as successful creatures on earth—our mind, with its unique ability to abstract, calculate, plan, diagnose—is in some way in decline for most of our lives. But this decline is normal; it is not dementia. To understand the decline for what it is—not a disease, and normal for age—is a comfort. If viewed from a certain perspective, it may appear that the cognitive arc is purposefully shaped, that even in old age the mind is devising some advantage that is overlooked in the youthful admiration for speedy, efficient, concrete productivity. There is, in fact, a bright side to cognitive aging. We will consider it in the next chapter, "Thinking Good Thoughts."

🔔 REMEMBER:

- ✓ Brains change. They grow, and they decline. Brain change is normal, and it is inevitable.

- ✓ Fluid intelligence (short-term recall, rapid information processing, pattern recognition) peaks in adolescence.

- ✓ By age 20, the parts of the brain that support fluid intelligence have fully matured but then begin to decline and will continue to do so into old age.

✓ In contrast, crystallized intelligence (skills, abilities, and knowledge that are learned, practiced, familiar and depend on experience, judgment, and wisdom) peaks in middle age.

✓ The prefrontal cortex (PFC) matures in middle age. The late maturation of the PFC helps sustain crystallized intelligence in middle age and after.

✓ Nevertheless, cognitive power declines after middle age. This decline is expected and is a normal part of brain aging.

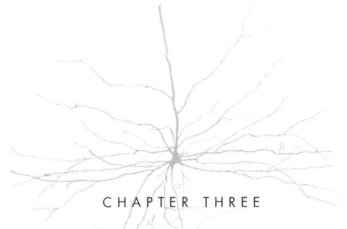

THINKING GOOD THOUGHTS: THE POSITIVE SIDE OF COGNITIVE AGING

On March 13, 2020, Judy Woodruff, of the *PBS Newshour*, spoke with her weekly guests, Mark Shields and David Brooks, about the beginning of the Covid-19 pandemic. In January, the CDC confirmed the first case of Covid-19 in the USA and the World Health Organization declared a global public health emergency. In February, global air travel was restricted and the CDC announced an imminent public health emergency. In March the WHO declared a pandemic. Judy Woodruff turned to Mark Shields.

> **Woodruff:** Where are we? How do you make sense of what's going on right now?
>
> **Shields:** The only way I can make sense of it is by what we've been through before. I'd compare it to the time right after World War II began, or the polio epidemic in the 50s…Especially after the beginning of the war it was a time of collective sacrifice. There were shortages of

alcohol, tobacco, meat, butter, you name it. But Americans, through 20 million Victory Gardens, raised one-third of America's vegetables, they saved tin, they sacrificed collectively. The president of the New York Stock Exchange went into the army: $21 a month, as a private, William McChesney Martin, later the chairman of the Federal Reserve. And at the time of polio there was terror in the country. I mean, we closed bowling alleys and swimming pools and beaches in the summer. 497,000 Americans were paralyzed. And then that magical moment in 1955 when there was a cure. That's where we are. It's the unknown. There's a sense of terror.

[Judy Woodruff turns to David Brooks.]

Woodruff: Can we make sense of it, David?

Brooks: Well, there are two issues, and maybe I should deal with them separately. One is the political and leadership issue, and one is the moral and social issue…

In real time, Mark Shield's statement is short, but it is dense with detail. He spontaneously recalls items that were unavailable in WWII, a wartime private's monthly Army salary, the fear of shared water that was part of society's experience of polio, the number of people paralyzed by polio and year the vaccine was first available. It is a statement rich with experience and memory. It brings a long perspective to a new problem. Mr. Shields' statement is the kind of well-told and vivid story that comes from a well-crystalized intelligence informed by long experience.

Mr. Brooks, in contrast, gets immediately to the point. He parses the subject into two issues, each of which, in turn, has two parts. He sees the logic of the problem and already has an outlined answer in mind. His entire statement is not included here, but it is concise yet thorough, precise in word choice yet fluent, and expressed with the confidence of a master of language who knows that any word he needs, however obscure, is within his grasp at any moment. His statement is less rangy, more focused, and a better example of fluid intelligence's concision and organizational power than the elder Mr. Shield's somewhat rambling explanation, which does not even mention the subject in question, Covid-19.

Both approaches to answering Judy Woodruff's open-ended questions are effective. Is one better than the other? Would someone charged with making important decisions prefer the counsel of one expert over the other?

Being organized, clear, concise, and speedy in the processing of information is valuable. But isn't there more to human intelligence? Depth is needed, a long view of consequences, and a comparison of historical similarities and differences. "The only way I can make sense of it," says Mark Shields, "is by what we've been through before." Experiential detail matter, and while a young, fluid mind is adept at assimilating many pieces of a puzzle into a meaningful whole, fluid intelligence has its limitations. In the first chapter of this book, fluid intelligence is described as the "problem-solving and reasoning about things that are less familiar and are independent of what one has learned." Fluid intelligence, by definition, is "independent of what one has learned." This is a plus and a minus. The young mind works like a computer processing unit that lacks data. Experience gives the mind character, strength, insight, and wisdom. Experience transforms raw, fluid intelligence into a capable mind. Events and experience connect, build, reinforce—crystalize—into a mind of clarity, durability, flexibility, and wisdom.

The neuropsychologic literature speaks of the "scaffolding theory of aging and cognition," or STAC. The theory observes that younger brains, when heavily taxed, use not just the prefrontal cortex (PFC) on the left side of the brain but on both sides. When a difficult task is practiced, and the cognitive circuitry becomes honed and efficient, the young brain no longer needs the power of both PFCs and falls back on use of the left prefrontal cortex alone. However, as the aging brain works begins to work more slowly and less efficiently in other ways, both PCFs are more frequently used. This is why, in part, older brains can still be effective brains. The PFCs compensate for the inefficiencies of other brain operations. They are like scaffolds propping up brain function. One author states:

> In the context we are using this term, scaffolding is a process that results in changes in brain function through strengthening of existing connections, formation of new connections, and disuse of connections that have become weak or faulty… Scaffolding is a process that characterizes neural dynamics across the lifespan…We view the recruitment of neural scaffolds as a normal adaptive response of the brain that takes place throughout the lifespan.[1]

In the STAC model, the use of the prefrontal cortex on both sides of the brain is more than just compensatory. The brain has expectations for itself. It has ambition and intention. It has a goal. Ever the good student, the brain struggles to improve itself, continually practicing and evolving. Encountering the stumbling block of neuronal decline in middle and late age, the

---

[1] Park DC, Reuter-Lorenz P. The Adaptive Brain: Aging and Neurocognitive Scaffolding. *Annu Rev Psychol* 2009;60: 173–196. DOI: 10.1146/annurev.psych.59.103006.093656

brain side-steps, takes a breath, re-arranges its operating system, leans increasingly on both PFCs for maintenance of function, and keeps moving toward a more perfect union of its parts.

What if the evolving brain has a particular mind in mind? What if scaffolding results not only in cognitive preservation but a specific kind of intelligence—an intelligence unique to older brains? It would be a kind of intelligence that—due to the inevitable decline of fluid intelligence—expresses its ideas slowly and with some word-finding pauses but still produces thoughtful, rational ideas by invoking a lifetime of vocabulary, cultural knowledge, and examples drawn from history and personal experience. What if Mark Shield's brain is the goal of cognitive aging?

The mistake we make in our understanding of the aged (please see footnote[2] for a comment on nomenclature) is the same automatic error we commit in judging the appearance of others: we assume that their outside reflect their insides. Mark Shields is jowly, his eyes baggy, his neck heavily wattled; he looks a lot like an owl. If you saw him waiting for a bus, for instance, and staring blankly at the street you would think him dull—if you noticed him at all among the other overlooked aged. You might, if his face held your attention for a moment longer, wonder what he might possibly have looked like as a young man—it is hard to tell with a face like Mark Shields'. In *An American Childhood*, Annie Dillard

---

[2] Some dignified synonyms for "old" are "aged" or "elderly." I prefer "old" because it is straightforward and specific. Most of the time, however, this book follows the preference of my mother-in-law who is over 80 years old and winces when called "old." She prefers "aged," "because it means a process." "Elderly," on the other hand, "means you're there." Other synonyms such as mature, senior, or ancient are unacceptable.

describes her childhood perspective on the aged. The revulsion she feels at the visible effects of age is natural, as if life itself, so strong in the child, is oil to aging's water.

> We children had, for instance, proper hands; our fluid, pliant fingers joined their skin. Adults had misshapen, knuckled hands loose in their skin like bones in bags; it was a wonder they could open jars. They were loose in their skins all over, except at the wrist and ankles, like rabbits.
>
> We were whole, we were pleasing to ourselves. Our crystalline eyes shone from firm, smooth sockets; we spoke in pure, piping voices through dark, tidy lips. Adults were coming apart...

The child is repelled by adults' sagging physicality. Skin droops, joints bulge, wattles waggle, voices weaken, eyes dim. There is disgust in Dillard's observation, as if adults, having allowed themselves to become misshapen, worsen their offense by failing to conceal it. I remember my own childish aversion to elderly bodies in swimsuits: the sight of their baggy frailty stimulated a mild electric shiver in my torso. Their insides, it seemed, must be as corroded and soft as their sagging outsides, and my shiver anticipated falls, easily broken bones, and the site of beached bodies on slick poolside cement with limbs at sickening angles. Yet even the child in Dillard's quotation sees through the bags of bones to a separate virtue, something quite apart from the degenerate bodies.

> ...We could never rise to the absolute figural splendor [adults] alone could on occasion achieve. Our beauty was a mere absence of decrepitude; their beauty, when they had it, was not passive but earned; it was

grandeur; it was a party to power, and to artifice, even, and to knowledge. Our beauty was, in the long run, merely elfin. We could not, finally, discount the fact that in some sense they owned us, and they owned the world.

Aging adults, coming apart bodily, nevertheless have beauty, gravity, and power. Their outsides and insides are mismatched, the former flaccid, the latter's splendor derived from earned experience and knowledge. The body declines, but the brain has an advantage not shared by other tissues such as skin, eyes, hair, muscle, lung. The brain—as demonstrated in STAC hypothesis of aging—takes aging's own momentum and redirects it, for a time, to bolster its power and even to make something new and powerful, something quite different from the young brain. The aged's crumbling exterior belies the firmer internal scaffolding of an effective mind.

"All processes of development entail both gains and losses."[3] Smooth skin is traded for gravitas, and the speedy, youthful brain is shed for something different but worthwhile. The brain moves on from its deterioration and continues to develop, evolve, and mature. Some changes are losses: loss of speed, loss of ready memory for new details and the fine, quick work of the mind. Some changes are gains: experience, judgement, sympathy, the ability to see the long view. Fluid knowledge, so useful early in life, gives way to crystalized knowledge. You cannot have, at the same time, the strength of crystalized knowledge and the flexibility of fluid knowledge. Time makes the choice for us.

---

[3] Craik FIM, Bialystok E. Cognition through the lifespan: mechanisms of change. *TRENDS in Cognitive Sciences* 2006;10(3). DOI: 10.1016/j.tics.2006.01.007

The Bible tells the story of two men: one builds his house on a rock, while the other builds on sand. The man who builds his house on a rock is said to be wise, the other foolish. The parable, however, is too simple and must be turned inside out to reflect the truth of cognitive aging. When we are young we are quick and smart, but we are foolish. "You are pretty and you are fast," says the old Grandfather Bunny in *The Country Bunny and the Little Golden Slippers* of the young rabbits vying for his approval, "but you have not shown me that you are either kind or wise." When we are older, we are slower, but we see, and we know. We sympathize and understand—even as our brains are in decline. The man is still foolish when he builds his house on a rock, and he becomes wise as his foundation turns to sand.

"There is no stable 'endstate' that the organism aspires to; rather, the continuing dynamics allow the possibility of growth and change at all stages of life, although different factors are dominant at different ages."[4] Instead of seeing decline, we can think of our mind as a project. We may not always like the way our project is going. It can be frustrating to have a word on the tip of the tongue but out of reach. Your child will recall the characters' names in a movie you watched together, yet you cannot even remember the movie's title. But your presence while watching the movie was probably still useful in clarifying relationships or contextualizing plot in a specific historic moment of which your child was not aware. We cannot change the aging of our minds, but we can choose to see the value in it.

---

[4] *Ibid*

Consider this description of Alexander Hamilton (his "young, crystalline eyes shining from firm, smooth sockets") by Joseph Ellis, in *The Quartet: Orchestrating the Second American Revolution, 1783-1789*:

> All came to regard him as a prodigy...He dazzled his employers with his deftness at manipulating account books and his conspicuous competence as a thirteen-year-old clerk...[He had a] trademark Hamilton style: an assurance bordering on arrogance; a slashing mode of attack that would one day make him the most feared polemicist in America; the capacity to control and incisively convey a large body of information...His defining characteristic was the ability to mesmerize everyone in his presence with the speed and flow of his conversation, which was simultaneously dazzling and yet never theatrical in an overly ostentatious fashion...The only conclusion to reach is that those resources [within himself] were truly massive...

Hamilton had an extraordinary fluid intelligence. He would have been an effective operator in any country in the world. He was sent by his benefactors to the British colonies in America, but had he been sent to India, he would have learned the local languages and thrived there, too. Yet although his brain was a powerful processor of information, he lacked wisdom. He had questionable real-life judgement, as demonstrated by his actions as a father, husband, and soldier, and in the manner of his death. Consider now this statement by Benjamin Franklin, age 81, upon signing the US Constitution:

> I confess that I do not entirely approve this Constitution at present, but Sir, I am not sure that I shall never approve it: For having lived long, I have experienced many Instances of being oblig'd, by better

Information or fuller Consideration, to change opinions on important Subjects, which I once thought Right, but found to be otherwise. It is therefore that the older I grow, the more apt I am to doubt my own Judgment, and to pay more respect to the Judgment of others.

Franklin calmly considers the facts of the Constitution from the perspective of a long life that included many successes, much experience, and abundant failures. Particularly poignant is his remarkable acceptance of others' judgement as equal to his own, a cognitive capacity that, perhaps more than any other, marks a mature mind. The ability to see both sides of a question and truly accept them as equally worthy of consideration seems a simple trick but is so rare among modern humans as to seem unnatural.

It is astonishing to read Franklin's statement in light of modern American politics. It seems that everywhere are Hamiltons, the quick-minded, the judgmental, the ferocious partisans with their "slashing mode of attack." Where are the Franklins? Have we mistaken their age for infirmity and retired them from public life? Would we have taken Franklin's aged face—so oddly similar to Mark Shields'—and his physical debility (Franklin was carried from Constitution Hall on a stretcher) to indicate worthlessness? His colleagues, young and old, made no such error. The framers needed Franklin; we, too, need Franklins. We need their perspective and years. We need their calm, their modesty, their experience, and their insight into the profound unimportance of their own beliefs and wishes. We need their ability to "pay more respect to the Judgment of others."

One wonders who was happier, Hamilton or Franklin. It is an easy guess. Hamilton died young and did not have the opportunity to experience the pleasures of a well-crystalized 81-year-old mind. For it is possible that a consequence of cognitive aging is a kind of contentment. Neurons are trimmed away, revealing the longer view. The mind is becalmed. "Older adults," maintain researchers of aging, emotion, and cognition, "prioritize emotional goals while younger adults pursue knowledge and information as they develop careers and become acquainted with the world."[5] Gone are youthful restlessness, searching, wanting. The subsiding anatomy of the aging mind may, in fact, be the anatomy of a kind of well-being. We will explore this possibility, in a different context, in chapter 10, "Is it So Bad to be Demented?."

[5] Knight BG, Durbin K. Aging and the effects of emotion on cognition: Implications for psychological interventions for depression and anxiety. *Psych J* 2015;4(1):11–19. DOI:10.1002/pchj.84

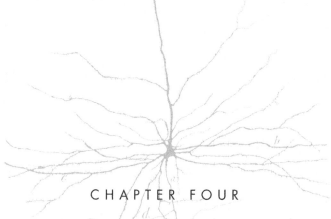

CHAPTER FOUR

ABNORMAL FOR AGE

"I've done something bad."

A friend was calling to confess. His voice shook on the telephone. I expected to hear about an infidelity or felony, but the real crime was endearingly human. He had taken a memory test and failed.

His sister was in her 50s and had been diagnosed with early-onset Alzheimer's disease. My friend, whom I will call Matt, was also in his 50s. Worried that he might also develop Alzheimer's at a young age, he completed a free online cognitive test and the results scared him. He had always been quick with math, but his mind had slowed in the last several years, and he was a little more forgetful. Did he, too, have Alzheimer's disease?

► The ability to assess the function of one's own mind is called "metacognition." People who report memory trouble are making a metacognitive assessment of their cognitive abilities.

► People who report memory trouble have Subjective Memory Complaints (SMCs), which are common and are reported by people of all ages.

► Dementia is unlikely in younger people with memory symptoms. After age 65, dementia risk increases.

► Mild Cognitive Impairment may be diagnosed when a person has subjective memory complaints accompanied by abnormal performance on memory testing.

► *Read on to learn more.*

1. METACOGNITION

The worry that Matt had for his mind is probably familiar to anyone reading this book. Matt felt that something could be wrong, but he did not know whether the problem was dementia or just excessive worry. Having memory symptoms can be normal. But when is forgetfulness abnormal?

It is telling that Matt didn't start the conversation by saying something like, "I think I have dementia." His first statement to me—"I've done something bad"—indicated a wider grasp of his predicament. He worried about dementia but he also knew that his worry could be pointless. Couldn't his amount of forgetfulness just be normal aging? Furthermore, he had taken a memory test, but he did not know if it was a good test. Were the results accurate and reliable? And finally, he knew that he was the kind of person whose health fears are easily triggered—he took the memory test against his better judgement. In short, he had done "something bad" because he was now stuck with a dilemma: was the problem in his brain, in the test, in his own excessive worry—or did he even have a problem at all?

Matt's skepticism was appropriate. Our insight into the status of our own minds is not always accurate. Cognitively normal people can misunderstand the competence of their own minds, believing them to be better or worse than they really are.

The ability to assess the competence of one's own mind is called "metacognition." It is the brain's ability to observe itself and make judgements about how it is operating. Metacognitive tasks are performed automatically and unconsciously, though we may be consciously aware of the results. When you are asked, for instance, whether you remember everything you need to buy at the store, you make a metacognitive assessment of the likelihood of recalling the list. Or another example, from the TV series *Breaking Bad*, in a scene in which the police are questioning a suspect—who has a limited memory but healthy metacognition—about the name of another suspect:[1]

Suspect: Mel. The dude's name was Mel.

Police: Mel who? Does he have a last name?

Suspect: Yeah, uh, Mel. Wait. Was it Mel, or Mark? It was definitely an "M" name. Oh, man, I'm losing it. Wait…wait…Yeah…It's gone!… It's gone…It was an "M" name though. I remember the "muh" sound.

Police: All right, well, we'll go with the "muh" sound.

Suspect: He definitely had tan pants.

Here we see the action of metacognition in real time. The suspect has a feeling that he knows the other suspect's name. He prompts himself ("It was definitely an 'M' name") and he thinks his memory has grasped it, but then his more competent metacognition steps in and questions the reliability of his memory ("Was it Mel, or Mark?"). His memory isn't dependable, and his metacognition knows it. His metacognition then watches the memory decay as the suspect narrates aloud the sensation of awareness of forgetting ("I'm losing it. Wait…wait…Yeah…It's gone.").

The actual sensation of metacognition's operation—the feeling of your mind scanning its memory when asked if you will remember a shopping list—is comprised of several more specific memory sensations. Most people would agree that they experience

---

[1] *Breaking Bad,* 3rd season, episode 4

these feelings, though they may have never directly acknowledged them, so intrinsic are they to the quick and familiar task of memory recovery. One such sensation is the "Feeling-of-Knowing," which is the intuitive sense of the contents of one's own memory. Feeling-of-Knowing (FOK) can occur "when one fails to retrieve specific information, and this feeling indicates the extent to which the information seems available in memory for future retrieval."[2] FOK is the feeling one has when the mind is reaching for a memory that it is senses is there but just out of reach, like in the case of the suspect, above, grasping for a name. FOKs indicate the likelihood that the target memory is somewhere in the mind. It is the feeling that people have when they say something is on the "tip of my tongue." The keener the FOK, the greater the urgency to grasp the nearly recovered thing, thus generating self-prompts like, "I know her name starts with a K," or "It's the same actor as was in…," or the *Breaking Bad* suspect remembering "the 'muh' sound." We rely on FOKs to give us a sense of what our memory contains.[3]

---

[2] Perrotin A, et al. Metamemory monitoring in mild cognitive impairment: Evidence of a less accurate episodic feeling-of-knowing. *Neuropsychologia* 2007;45:2811–2826. DOI: 10.1016/j.neuropsychologia.2007.05.003

[3] There is a difference between Feeling-of-Knowing events—a term used to describe a neurologic phenomenon associated with the act of memory recovery—and the feeling one has that something is true. FOKs are a product of our cognitive machinery and give a sense of the probability that a memory is in the mind or not. However, in another kind of feeling of knowing, the target concept is outside the mind, for example, one's feelings about the truthfulness of a politician's statement, the reality of global warming, a virus' potential harm, or the existence of deities. The truth value of this kind of feeling of knowing is nil. The intuition that the earth is or is not warming does not change the likelihood of the event. An individual's feeling that gods exist does not count as proper proof to anyone else. The truth value of neurologic FOKs is confined to what is or is not contained in one's own memory and have no application to facts existing outside one's own mind.

The point of including metacognition and feeling-of-knowing in this discussion of memory complaints is to give a nuts-and-bolts sense of how we perceive the functioning of our own minds. Built into our brains are the mechanisms for monitoring how the brain itself is functioning. Sometimes these mechanisms work well, accurately informing us of mistakes, and sometimes they don't. They can even lead us astray about how well our brains are operating. Metacognition and feeling-of-knowing are like sensors in a machine (a dishwasher, for example, or car) that monitor temperature, electrical current, or pressure and sound an alarm when something breaks or needs adjustment. If a sensor is set for a very wide temperature range, it will rarely trigger: things must go very wrong for the engine to overheat outside the range and set off the alarm. But if the acceptable temperature range is set very narrowly then it will be easily exceeded, and the alarm will be triggered more often.

Metacognition works the same way. If the function of a person's memory has a wide range of "normal" (if a generous number of memory mistakes can be made without triggering an alarm), then a person will not have a sense of abnormal memory performance. If, on the other hand, metacognition's normal range is set very narrowly—it's alarm easily and frequently triggered— then the person will believe that their memory is abnormal. This person will also probably interpret their memory failures as ominous and abnormal. Moreover, once a person becomes aware of memory mistakes (whether normal for age or not), metacognition may re-calibrate or re-sensitize itself; it becomes increasingly focused on identifying error, noting even the mildest mis-firings, like a temperature sensor whose range of normal has become too narrow and its alarm triggered so frequently that normal operation becomes impossible. The machine becomes paralyzed in monitoring its own errors.

Consider again Matt, whose sister's dementia diagnosis made him worry for his own mind. He had a top-notch graduate degree and the kind of job that defines the term "successful business executive." His colleagues and clients appeared in the news. His work was busy, he travelled often, and he had many projects in play at once. In short, he had an excellent memory, superior executive function,[4] was a quick and flexible learner, and was at the peak of his cognitive abilities with a well-crystalized intelligence. His metacognition perceived a change in the reliability of his fluid intelligence, and this caused him to worry that his memory was not as reliable as it should be. But it is possible that his metacognition mislead him, and that his brain otherwise functioned normally. Perhaps his high standards for himself imposed unrealistically severe expectations for his mind. Or perhaps his metacognition became over-focused on error, shrinking the range of acceptable error such that his metacognitive alarm became too sensitive, informing him too often that something was wrong. Matt feared that the explanation for these metacognitive alarms was early-onset dementia. But his symptoms—particularly in the context of his young age and normal work performance—may be better explained by normal cognitive aging plus the disabling effects of worry.

---

[4] Recall from chapter 2 that executive function is "a set of higher order cognitive processes including the monitoring and control of behavior, planning, inhibition of irrelevant information, shifting." EF is the brain overseeing itself. The prefrontal cortex is the center for executive function, and its role in brain oversight also extends to monitoring the reliability of memory formation.

There are, therefore, three important truths to remember about metacognition. First, metacognition's purpose is to tell us how our brains are operating. Second, metacognition may become over-sensitized to memory mistakes. And third, metacognitive feedback is not always accurate. Sometimes metacognition over-estimates what is held in one's memory, identifying a memory as intact when it is not. Sometimes metacognition does the opposite, erroneously detecting a significant memory failure when no such failure has occurred. A study of 75-year-olds found no difference in cognitive abilities between those who complained about their memory and those who did not, telling us that metacognitively accurate memory complaints are not readily distinguished from metacognitive errors.[5] Does an awareness of memory decline hold any truth value—does it reliably predict dementia? How would Matt know if his sense of cognitive doom was accurate, or whether he was just worried? When a person says that they have memory problems, they have "Subjective Memory Complaints,", which are the crossroads of normal and abnormal cognition.

2. SUBJECTIVE MEMORY COMPLAINTS

When an individual reports memory trouble, they have, by definition, "Subjective Memory Complaints," or SMCs. ("Subjective" in this case indicates that the complaints have not been supported by more objective memory testing.) SMCs are present when the answer to any of the following sort of questions is "yes":

------

[5] Jungwirth S, et al. Subjective Memory Complaints and Objective Memory Impairment in the Vienna-Transdanube Aging Community. *JAGS* 2004 52:263–268

Do you think you have trouble with your memory?

In general, do you feel your memory is abnormal for a person your age?

In general, do you feel you remember things less well than you did a year ago?

Do you feel like your memory is becoming worse?

Do you feel as if you have any problems with any aspect of your thinking or memory lately?

Many people answer "yes" to at least one of these questions. A Dutch study asked people of all ages, "Do you consider yourself forgetful?" and 38% said "yes." Half of the oldest people in this study (ages 70-85) acknowledged forgetfulness, but so did 29% of 25-35-year-olds and 33.9% of 40-50-year-olds.[6]

So, it seems that if you ask a group of adults of any age, "Do you consider yourself forgetful?" a substantial percentage will answer "yes." People have a low threshold to acknowledging forgetfulness, and many factors, besides dementia, affect people's perception of their memory.

The reliability of self-reported memory complaints is not high. For instance, one study compared older people's memory complaints with results of objective cognitive testing.[7] 39% of them admitted memory problems. These results are not unexpected—we develop memory trouble as we age—but it is interesting that

---

[6] Commissaris CJAM, et al. Subjective forgetfulness in a normal Dutch population: possibilities for health education and other interventions. *Patient Education and Counseling* 1998;34:25–32

[7] Jungwirth S, et al. Subjective Memory Complaints and Objective Memory Impairment in the Vienna-Transdanube Aging Community. *JAGS* 2004. 52:263–268

some people had little insight into their actual memory capabilities. "Only 6.3% of the subjects who scored [significantly lower] than the mean of the age cohort in a memory test also complained about their memory." Furthermore, "9.1% of subjects with memory performance [significantly] above the mean also complained about their memory." Stated differently, some patients complained about their memory, yet their brains worked very well, while other felt that their memory was normal but it was not.

Matt had subjective memory complaints. He believed that his memory was not what it should have been. It is right to be concerned about one's memory if there is cause, if memory mistakes occur regularly, and particularly if they interfere with normal function. (And particularly after age 65, when the likelihood of dementia substantially increases.) But the line between mere memory complaints and true cognitive dysfunction is often unclear to the person with the memory symptoms. Matt had a hunch, but despite his good overall cognitive competence he was unable to know if he was cognitively abnormal or just worried.

The point is that many cognitive normal people have memory symptoms. Memory symptoms may be present at any age, may be unrelated to neurologic disease, and may occur in healthy, normal people. In sorting out whether memory symptoms are normal or abnormal for age, we cannot rely on the memory symptoms themselves. We need somehow to double-check an individual's metacognitive impressions. We need bring something objective to the problem, something that can help distinguish normal memory function from dementia-related dysfunction.

That "something objective" is found in the criteria for a widely used diagnosis, Mild Cognitive Impairment. A diagnosis of Mild

Cognitive Impairment (MCI) means that cognition is abnormal according to the individual or their family (they report having subjective memory complaints). But it requires something extra: abnormal results on cognitive testing. Using objective data (cognitive testing) plus subjective memory complaints increases MCI's reliability in identifying people whose cognition is truly abnormal. Conversely, having subjective memory complaints with normal cognitive testing means that dementia is very unlikely. Applying the MCI criteria to an individual's memory issues is an important step is sorting normal forgetfulness from abnormal.

Mild Cognitive Impairment is usually considered as a transitional phase between normal cognition and dementia, because having MCI increases the chance that dementia will develop. The diagnosis is widely accepted as a trustworthy tool in identifying patients at risk for dementia. In the next chapter, we will examine MCI (and its drawbacks) in more detail.

Some months after our conversation about his memory, I asked Matt how he was doing. He did not want to talk. His sister's health had declined, and Matt was involved in her care. The tragedy of his sister's case probably exacerbated his worry for himself, which had grown despite a neurologic evaluation that did not result in a diagnosis of dementia (in fact, he performed normally on subsequent cognitive testing—he did not have Mild Cognitive Impairment). Matt was caught in the "vicious circle of distress, cognitive dysfunction, anxiety, and frustration [that] may be set in motion" and exacerbate subjective memory complaints, a process likely enhanced when true neurologic disease is witnessed in a family member.[8] He was hyper-vigilant of his cognitive mistakes, thus hampering normal memory function and de-calibrating his metacognition such that even talking with me about his symptoms presented yet another occasion for disruptive self-scrutiny.

Some people, like Matt, who have harmful subjective memory complaints and a family history of dementia, need more and better information about their true dementia risk. In fact, a person's perception of the risk for dementia is often quite different than the actual risk—as we will learn in chapter 7, "What a Family History of Dementia Means for You."

🔔 REMEMBER:

✓ "Metacognition" is the brain's ability to monitor its own cognitive processes.

✓ People who say they have memory trouble are making a metacognitive assessment of their cognitive abilities.

✓ People's metacognitive impressions are not always accurate. Some people believe that their memory errors indicate a problem, but they may be mistaken.

---

[8] Schmidtke K, et al. The Syndrome of Functional Memory Disorder: Definition, Etiology, and Natural Course. *Am J Geriatr Psychiatry* 2008;16:981–988

✓ People who report memory trouble are acknowledging Subjective Memory Complaints (SMCs).
SMCs are common and are reported by people
of all ages.

✓ Having subjective memory complaints does not
always mean that one has dementia. Cognitively normal people report SMCs, as do demented
individuals.

✓ It is unlikely that memory complaints before age
65 are due to dementia.

✓ Mild Cognitive Impairment (MCI) may be diagnosed when a person has subjective memory complaints plus abnormal memory testing.

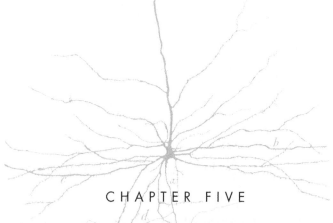

CHAPTER FIVE

MILD COGNITIVE IMPAIRMENT

So you forgot a few things. They weren't important things, just little things. It's not like you forgot to pick the kids up from school. But... Once you even forgot what you forgot. You were talking to someone and trying to remember the name of a movie, and then you forgot what you were trying to remember. Embarrassing.

So what? People forget stuff. It happens with age. It's nothing like dementia. You don't need help with eating and dressing.

You tell yourself that you haven't been sleeping well. You take a sleep aid and it helps, but then you're groggy the next morning. Your sleep would be better if you could exercise, but work has been too busy and you don't have time for that. Work is really stressful and you feel like you can never put it aside. You're always thinking about work. And how could you have dementia if you're still able to work? No one at work has commented about a problem, you're doing fine there. But at home there have been comments about your memory.

Forgetfulness can progress such that it becomes more obvious to you or others in your family. This may still be normal for age. And it is true that non-neurologic factors can worsen normal forgetfulness: poor sleep, anxiety, depression, work preoccupation, excessive alcohol use, medications, and other treatable problems. But when formal cognitive testing is abnormal—suggesting a diagnosis of Mild Cognitive Impairment—then dementia is a possibility.

► Mild Cognitive Impairment (MCI) is diagnosed when a person has cognitive difficulties that are confirmed on formal cognitive testing.

► Each year, a small percentage of people with MCI are diagnosed with dementia.

► Most people with MCI either do not progress to dementia or their cognitive function normalizes.

► A diagnosis of Mild Cognitive Impairment should prompt a neurologic workup, but there is no treatment for MCI.

► *Read on to learn more.*

1. MILD COGNITIVE IMPAIRMENT

Mild Cognitive Impairment (MCI) occupies the vexed territory between normal cognition and dementia. MCI is diagnosed when a patient or family report cognitive difficulties that are confirmed on formal memory testing, yet without associated impairment of normal daily activities. A neurologist, Ronald Peterson, describes the features of MCI in the *New England Journal of Medicine*:

> Typically, [people with MCI] start to forget important information that they previously would have remembered easily, such as appointments, telephone conversations, or recent events that would normally interest them (e.g., for a sports fan, outcomes of sporting events). However, virtually all other aspects of function are preserved. The forgetfulness is generally apparent to those close to the person but not to the casual observer.[1] [2]

Younger people with subjective memory complaints are unlikely to have MCI, but by age 65 the prevalence of MCI is 10-20%. While age is the strongest risk factor for MCI, other risks are the number of cognitive complaints (the more cognitive complaints, the more likely they are due to MCI), cardiovascular problems such as high blood pressure and heart disease, as well as diabetes, high cholesterol, and a family history of dementia.[3] [4]

[1] Ronald Peterson was one of the first researchers to characterize MCI, in the 1990s

[2] Peterson R. Mild Cognitive Impairment. *N Engl J Med* 2011;364:2227-34

[3] Clement F, et al. Cognitive complaint in mild cognitive impairment and Alzheimer's disease. *Journal of the International Neuropsychological Society.*2008;14, 222–232. DOI: 10.10170S1355617708080260

[4] We will discuss some of these risk factors further in later chapters, and we will specifically examine the risks posed by a family history of dementia in Chapter 7, "What a Family History of Dementia Means for You."

Mild Cognitive Impairment is considered a step in the wrong direction, a transition between normal cognition and dementia. One researcher declares that "MCI should be recognized as part of a spectrum, with normal cognition on 1 end of the spectrum and dementia on the other end."[5] Rate of progression from MCI to dementia is approximately 5-10% per year, while yearly incidence of dementia for cognitively normal individuals (of comparable age) is only 1-2%.

These are the facts that we must live with. Once forgetfulness reaches a certain point, dementia is possible. That "certain point" of higher dementia risk requires two elements: subjective memory complaints plus abnormal results on cognitive testing. Having only subjective memory complaints does not pose the same risk for dementia as when cognitive testing is abnormal. To illustrate this difference in risk, let's return to the case of Carol and her mother, Millie, whom we met in an earlier chapter. Millie lives with Carol and is now 80 years old. She has been forgetful for some time—but so has Carol. Do they share a diagnosis?

Carol or Millie: Who has Mild Cognitive Impairment?

Millie forgets day-to-day things. She forgot her appointment at the bank. But she remembered happy hour. She forgot to pick up her prescription but not her People *magazine. Maybe, Carol wonders, there is a pattern there. In her old age, is her mother just more relaxed, de-prioritizing things she doesn't*

---

[5] Sanford A. Mild Cognitive Impairment. *Clin Geriatr Med* 2017;33:25–337. DOI: 10.1016/j.cger.2017.02.005

care that much about? Or is she forgetful in a way that is worrisome? After all, Millie takes care of herself just fine. She doesn't need help with much. She has a well-tended garden. She often makes herself useful around the house. And Millie herself doesn't think there's anything wrong.

When she notices her mother's forgetfulness, Carol sometimes feels like the pot calling the kettle black. Because Carol forgets, too. Small stuff—like where she put her car keys after work. She forgot a website password—then remembered it. More troubling is the difficulty she sometimes has finding the right word. She knows the word she wants to say but can't put her finger on it. Today she couldn't remember the word "prospectus"—an unusual word, but she is a financial advisor it should have come easily to her.

Eventually, Carol takes her mother to the doctor under the pretense of adjusting her blood pressure medication. But what she really wants to talk about is her mother's memory. And she has a second covert agenda: she hopes to learn something about her own forgetfulness.

The doctor talks about Mild Cognitive Impairment, and Carol understands that to have this diagnosis a person (or their family member) must report forgetfulness. People with MCI are still able to do all the things they usually do like driving or shopping, says the doctor, but they don't score normally on memory testing. Millie denies forgetfulness, but Carol confirms for the doctor that Millie is forgetful.

The doctor gives Millie a memory test. Carol surreptitiously takes the test along with her mother. Millie doesn't do so well, and Carol's disappointment in her mother's result is mixed with relief at her own score, which is perfect. She feels something inside her relax. She didn't realize she was so worried, and she is surprised that this one small bit of objective information about her cognitive health gives her so much reassurance.

The doctor tells Millie that she has Mild Cognitive Impairment. MCI, the doctor says, is kind of a pre-condition to Alzheimer's disease. Having MCI increases the chance that Millie will develop dementia. The doctor orders some blood tests, and they schedule a follow-up visit to review the results.

Her mother takes in this information as a matter of course. Perhaps some of her friends have MCI, too, Carol thinks. Millie doesn't ask the doctor any questions about her diagnosis, but Carol is concerned. Based on the information from the doctor, dementia seems kind of inevitable for her mother, and Carol has questions. She is a numbers person, and she wants to know the actual odds. She wants to understand the details. She resolves to research MCI and dementia in preparation for her mother's follow-up with the doctor.

2. WHAT DOES A DIAGNOSIS OF MCI MEAN?

10-20% of people over age 65 have MCI, and the risk for progression from MCI to dementia is 5-10% per year. These numbers are well-established and reliable—yet skepticism about some aspects of the diagnosis is warranted. It is necessary to look closely at the assumptions and real implications behind MCI as a diagnosis. For although the statistics accurately reflect the tendencies of large groups, the reader of this book is not a group but an individual. How do these numbers apply to you?

The next few paragraphs examine two questions. The first is whether dementia is the inevitable outcome of Mild Cognitive Impairment. The second question asks whether MCI is a diagnosis that gives useful information to the individual.

In questioning these aspects of Mild Cognitive Impairment, the intention is not to deny that forgetfulness can be ominous or that MCI is a real and relevant diagnosis. Cognitive complaints must be taken seriously. The intention here is simply to offer an alternative perspective on medical science's consensus, which sees a glass 90% full and calls it empty. When we read of a 5-10% yearly conversion rate from MCI to dementia, it is natural for those of us concerned for our minds to ask the obvious question: If only 5-10% of MCI patients progress to dementia, what happens to the other 90-95%?

Good medical research answers specific questions. For example, instead of asking, "Does diet increase the risk for dementia?" a better question is: "Does a diet high in fats, and specifically polyunsaturated fats, increase the risk for vascular dementia?" This kind of focus increases the reliability of research findings. Using the diagnosis of Mild Cognitive Impairment in research helps to narrow down the kind of cognitive symptoms that are studied. It allows researchers to study groups of patients whose cognitive characteristics are defined by widely accepted criteria, thus creating consistency among studies and reliability in their findings.

We need researchers working on a cure for Alzheimer's disease, and Mild Cognitive Impairment is a tool for identifying patients at risk for AD. Most people with memory complaints, however, are not enrolled in clinical trials, and it is possible that the tail of MCI research is wagging the clinical dog. I disagree, for instance, that a diagnosis of MCI is a useful predictor of future cognitive welfare for an individual.

Published reviews of Mild Cognitive Impairment focus on the 5-10% of patients who progress each year to dementia. (Please see footnote[6] for more information about conversion rates.) But less is said about the two other groups consistently identified in MCI studies: those who "revert," becoming cognitively

---

[6] Higher yearly rates of conversion from MCI to dementia are cited in some publications, particularly in the early MCI literature, in which authors frequently assumed that MCI always led to dementia. However, rates of conversion quoted in the early MCI literature were often poorly supported by the cited sources, many of which were not studies of patients with MCI (as it was later defined), were small studies performed in the context of specialty memory clinics, did not follow patients over time, or, if they did, only followed them for a short time. Claims about MCI progression rates were eventually analyzed by a timely meta-analysis of the MCI literature (Mitchell AJ, Shiri-Feshki A. Rate of progression of mild cognitive impairment to dementia—meta-analysis of 41 robust inception cohort studies. *Acta Psychiatr Scand* 2009;119(4):252–65), which calculated an annual conversion rate from MCI to dementia of about 7%, stating that, "A 10–15% annual conversion rate has been very widely cited but rarely scrutinized using robust data...If a 10% annual conversion rate held true then within 10 years of diagnosis almost all surviving MCI suffers would have dementia...This has led many to suggest that MCI is an inescapable intermediate stage between normal ageing and dementia. Against this, it is well known that not all patients with MCI deteriorate. In fact some patients appear to improve over time."

normal for age and thus no longer qualifying as having MCI, and those "stable" subjects who neither progress nor revert. These two patient groups are as relevant to an individual attempting to understand their dementia risk as those that progress from Mild Cognitive Impairment to dementia, and they are also the majority: if 5-10% of people with MCI each year progress to dementia, then 90-95% do not.

But this is not how the scientific literature presents Mild Cognitive Impairment. In the 2011 review of MCI, cited above, one gets the sense that people with MCI are imminently demented, while an alternative to this inevitable progression is given a single sentence: "Although some data suggest that the rate of reversion to normal cognition may be as high as 25 to 30%, recent prospective studies have shown lower rates." The author is speaking of the percentage of MCI patients who do not progress to dementia but revert to normal. Yet other studies report higher reversion rates. One study (in which Peterson is listed as an author) found a 38% rate of reversion from MCI to normal, and a 2017 review of MCI identifies a 30-50% reversion rate.[7][8] A fair review of the MCI literature tells us that the rate of reversion to normal from MCI may be more than triple the rate of progression to dementia.

Thus far we have seen that a large percentage of Mild Cognitive Impairment cases revert to normal, while a small

---

[7] Geda YE, et al. Higher risk of progression to dementia in mild cognitive impairment cases who revert to normal, *Neurology* 2014 (82); 317–325

[8] Sanford A. Mild Cognitive Impairment. *Clin Geriatr Med* 2017;33:25–337. DOI: 10.1016/j.cger.2017.02.005

percentage progresses to dementia. Then there is the third MCI sub-group, the so-called "stable" patients who neither progress to dementia nor revert to normal. The literature demonstrates that this is the largest MCI sub-group of all, with 37-67% remaining cognitively stable over 1.5-5 years.[9] A journal article highlighting this ignored MCI group states that, "MCI stability rates are substantially higher than MCI reversion and progression rates, suggesting that MCI stability might be the most common observation after a diagnosis of MCI is established."[10]

Knowing this, one must question the assertion, quoted earlier, that "MCI should be recognized as part of a spectrum, with normal cognition on 1 end of the spectrum and dementia on the other end." "Spectrum" implies gradation, progression, a march from one state to another. Yet most people with a diagnosis of Mild Cognitive Impairment do not experience an inevitable downward slide. People

---

[9] Five years is a substantial percentage of this aged group's remaining lifespan. See the following references:

Artero S, et al. Risk profiles for mild cognitive impairment and progression to dementia are gender specific. *J Neurol Neurosurg Psychiatry* 79 (9) (2008) 979–984. DOI: 10.1136/ jnnp.2007.136903.

Manly JJ. Frequency and course of mild cognitive impairment in a multiethnic community. *Ann Neurology* 2008;63 (4):494–506. DOI: 10.1002/ana.21326.

Ravaglia G, et al. Mild cognitive impairment: epidemiology and dementia risk in an elderly Italian population. *J Am Geriatr Soc* 2008;56 (1): 51–58. DOI: 10.1111/ j.1532-5415.2007.01503.

Roberts RO, et al. Higher risk of progression to dementia in mild cognitive impairment cases who revert to nor- mal, *Neurology* 2014;82:317–325.

Sachdev PS, et al. Factors predicting reversion from mild cognitive impairment to normal cognitive functioning: a population-based study. *PLoS One* 2013;8(3):1–10.

[10] Pandya SY, et al. Does mild cognitive impairment always lead to dementia? A review. Journal of the Neurological Sciences 369 (2016) 57–62. DOI: 10.1016/j.jns.2016.07.055

with MCI are a cognitively diverse group whose membership is in flux, with many members normalizing and leaving the group, and many remaining in the MCI range without significant change either for the worse or the better. As noted by the authors of the paper Does Mild Cognitive Impairment Always Lead to Dementia?:

> A growing number of research groups have found high rates of MCI reversion and stability, each of which is frequently higher than that of MCI progression to dementia. These rates appear to remain high when followed over time, contradictory to the generally held notion that MCI is an intermediate stage between normal aging and inevitable dementia…Based on existing studies, progression to dementia from MCI is relatively and surprisingly rare. Given this, as well as its variable course, MCI appears to have poor predictive validity regarding future dementia, and does not always imply incipient Alzheimer's or other types of dementias.

Many people diagnosed with MCI are cognitively normal for age and it is a mistake, in my opinion, to suggest to them otherwise, for the following reasons.

Subjective memory complaints are unreliable. SMCs are a critical part of the criteria for mild cognitive impairment, but we have seen that a large percentage of people who complain about their memory are cognitively healthy. The risk that memory complaints indicate a true neurologic memory problem increases with age, but even among older patients with subjective memory complaints a substantial number do not have dementia.

A diagnosis of MCI lacks specificity. When diagnosed with MCI, a person joins a large and cognitively diverse group. The memory symptoms of most of the group—and particularly the younger members—are unrelated to neurologic disease but due to insomnia, depression, ruminative style, hypochondriasis, Alzheimer's phobia, medication side effects, chronic pain, excessive alcohol use, thyroid dysfunction, among other possibilities, or just to the predictable cognitive decline of normal aging.

The chance that Mild Cognitive Impairment will evolve into dementia is about 5-10% annually, which is very low, and it is doubtful whether a test of such poor predictive value would be considered useful in another context. Yet MCI is widely applied by physicians. This is especially odd considering the position that neurologists have taken on *APOE* genetic testing (which is discussed in detail in chapter 8). In brief, having one copy of the *APOE*4 gene increases the risk for Alzheimer's disease by 2-3 times, and two copies of the gene increases risk by a factor of 5-6. But because having the gene does not guarantee Alzheimer's disease, *APOE* testing is not recommended for the evaluation of patients with memory symptoms. Nevertheless, these same patients with memory complaints may be assigned a diagnosis of MCI, which entails an even lower likelihood for dementia (10-15%) than does the *APOE*4 gene.

There is a potential psychologic cost to assigning a patient a diagnosis of MCI. Receiving a diagnosis of Mild Cognitive Impairment may reduce the chance of stability and complicate the journey to reversion. Many MCI patients' concerns will be informed by pre-existing anxiety or other mood disorders, which may be exacerbated by an MCI diagnosis. "It is imperative," writes a researcher, "to begin to understand the impact of applying diagnostic labels to groups that have mild or even no symptoms."[11] Another author describes the feedback loop of worry encouraged by an MCI diagnosis:

> Life events or circumstances elicit long-term psychological and emotional distress...[causing] a state of internal distractedness, reduced ability to focus, to maintain attention, and slowing of thought processes...Reduced attention and distractibility can also lead to decreased short-term memory performance, causing instances of rapid forgetting, disruption of the coherence of thoughts, and failure to retain a task or errand while being on one's way to dispatch it...Deficits of memory and concentration can elicit objective problems in daily living, rumination, self-accusation, and fear of organic disease. Such objective and subjective consequences can amount to significant secondary stress factors. Thereby, a vicious circle of distress, cognitive dysfunction, anxiety, and frustration may be set in motion.[12]

In short, when some patients hear "Mild Cognitive Impairment", the words they will hear most clearly are "cognitive impairment"—even when their brains are normal.

A diagnosis of MCI does not change treatment. An older patient (65 or older) with memory complaints, whether they have objective memory dysfunction or not, needs a basic neurologic workup for dementia, including imaging and blood testing. Neuropsychologic

---

[11] Stites SD, et al. Awareness of Mild Cognitive Impairment and Mild Alzheimer's Disease Dementia Diagnoses Associated With Lower Self-Ratings of Quality of Life in Older Adults. *J Gerontol B Psychol Sci Soc Sci* 2017;72(6,):974–985. DOI:10.1093/geronb/gbx100

[12] Schmidtke K, et al. The Syndrome of Functional Memory Disorder: Definition, Etiology, and Natural Course. *Am J Geriatr Psychiatry* 2008;16:981–988

testing may be considered, too, depending on the nature of the cognitive complaint, the degree of worry that the symptom is causing, and whether modifiable factors (insomnia, medication side effects) are present. It is reasonable to consider this workup in all patients with memory trouble, whether or not they satisfy criteria for Mild Cognitive Impairment.

How then does a diagnosis of Mild Cognitive Impairment change a patient's treatment? Most serious diagnoses are followed by disease-specific treatments. Once diagnosed with Parkinson's disease, dopamine-enhancing medications improve patients' walking. A stroke triggers a unique workup and a variety of treatment alternatives. A diagnosis of multiple sclerosis opens very specific treatment options to the patient that are different than those recommended to people with seizures. Even non-ominous neurologic diagnoses entail specific treatments: migraine, restless leg syndrome, essential tremor, neuropathy, carpal tunnel syndrome each entail a unique treatment. Mild Cognitive Impairment is an exception. The workup of memory complaints would be the same whether the diagnosis of "Mild Cognitive Impairment" existed or not. And MCI is not treated with a specific memory medication, because "at present, no medication intended for the treatment of Mild Cognitive Impairment has been approved by the Food and Drug Administration."[13]

Consider this hypothetical. After many decades of research, a medication is at last developed that prevents Alzheimer's disease. It is quite expensive, of course, and it only works on patients who will definitely develop AD. Therefore, medical insurance

---

[13] Peterson R. Mild Cognitive Impairment. *N Engl J Med* 2011;364:2227-34

will only pay for the treatment in patients with a high probability of the disease. Let's also say that the medication must be
given preventively; it cannot reverse Alzheimer's disease once a
person has it. In this scenario, there is enormous pressure from
patients and families to give the preventive treatment before
the disease is diagnosed (for example, when a person has Mild
Cognitive Impairment), but there is an opposite pressure from
medical insurance not to give an expensive medication unneces-
sarily. Would it make sense to give the medication to everyone
diagnosed with MCI, knowing that only 5-10% of all patients
will progress each year to dementia, while 30-50% will revert to
normal and 37-67% will fail to progress? Market forces and the
edict to do no harm with unnecessary treatments make use of
this medication unlikely.

Is there an argument to be made in favor of using Mild Cognitive
Impairment as a diagnosis? We have seen that it is useful in
academic research, but are there other circumstances in which
MCI is useful? The answer is yes. Older patients with Mild
Cognitive Impairment and more cognitive symptoms are more
likely to progress to dementia, as are those with a family history of
dementia. Subjective Memory Complaints—one of the pillars on
which the MCI diagnosis is based—do not necessarily indicate
dementia, but they are important in that they get the patient into
the physician's office to begin a workup. From a purely practical standpoint, assigning an MCI diagnosis gives the physician
leverage with insurance companies to proceed with a neurologic
evaluation. This is what Millie's doctor did. Carol told the doctor

that Millie was forgetful. Memory testing in the doctor's office was abnormal, thus establishing a diagnosis of Mild Cognitive Impairment, and her doctor then ordered tests to evaluate for causes of forgetfulness. Giving Millie a diagnosis of MCI allowed her doctor to take steps in evaluating her symptoms.

Carol and Millie: The gift of stability

Millie's blood tests show that her liver, kidneys, and thyroid are functioning normally. Her vitamin B12 level is normal, as is her physical exam. The doctor says that there is no treatment for Mild Cognitive Impairment, and that Millie does not have dementia, so there is nothing further to do unless Millie's forgetfulness increases.

But over the next year, Millie's forgetfulness does not change. It does not worsen, and it does not really improve. She continues to do all the things she enjoys—seeing friends, gardening, talking on the telephone, playing solitaire on her computer, watching British TV. Carol, having researched Mild Cognitive Impairment, is relieved that her mother is among the 37-67% of people diagnosed with MCI who are "stable," neither progressing nor reverting to normal. Her mother's cognitive health may not remain stable forever, but Carol is thankful that her mother can continue to have a normal life for now.

And Carol is thankful that her own cognition has also stabilized. She still makes memory mistakes, but she is less concerned about them. Perhaps she had her fill of worry and just doesn't want to worry any more. Her guardedly optimistic feelings about her own cognitive welfare also may have something to do with mother's stable course: it seems unlikely to Carol that she will develop dementia if her mother does not. And her mind regularly returns to her perfect score on the memory test—a touchstone of reassurance for Carol. She makes a conscious effort to stay optimistic, for herself and for her mother.

Mild Cognitive Impairment encompasses a diverse group of patients with very different cognitive fates. Rather than a slope along which patients inevitably slip from normal to demented, the MCI cohort is better imagined as a flux. People enter the domain of MCI but many exit, and more will neither exit nor progress but reach a kind of cognitive equilibrium within the MCI range. A minority proceed on a more direct course from MCI to dementia. Let us step back and review the most important points discussed in this chapter.

1. **Most people with cognitive symptoms who** are younger than age 65 are neurologically normal. Our minds age. This is expected. Dementia is uncommon before age 65 but it does sometimes occur, and it is reasonable to look for all causes of cognitive decline—particularly if others confirm a memory problem. The most likely causes of cognitive difficulties in younger people are mood issues (anxiety, depression), insomnia, medication effects, or chronic pain—but not dementia.

2. **Subjective memory concerns are relevant.** Subjective memory complaints are a crossroads between normal and abnormal cognitive aging. Most people with SMCs do not have dementia. Subjective Memory Complaints serve as a starting point for an evaluation of cognitive symptoms.

3. **Mild Cognitive Impairment is defined as** subjective memory complaints plus abnormal cognitive testing, but without problems with activities of daily life (self-care, cooking, finances, shopping). MCI usually does not result in dementia: 90-95% of patients with the diagnosis do not progress within the next year to dementia, while the cognition of 25-35% of people with MCI will normalize.

4. **Factors that may increase the risk** of progression from MCI to dementia are higher age, cardiovascular disease, moderately to severely abnormal cognitive test results (in contrast to borderline or mildly abnormal results), or abnormalities on brain imaging.

5. **Factors that increase the chance of** "reversion" in Mild Cognitive Impairment are higher cognitive test scores, absence of memory problems reported by relatives of the person with memory complaints, depression (treatment may improve cognition), the use of medications that might cause forgetfulness, lower blood pressure, regular complex mental activity, and absence of the *APOE4* gene.

6. **Suspicion for true neurologic disease should** prompt further workup, including brain imaging, blood testing, and formal neuropsychologic testing.

🔔 REMEMBER:

✓ Mild Cognitive Impairment (MCI) is diagnosed when a person, or their family, reports cognitive difficulties that are confirmed on formal cognitive testing, yet independent living activities are preserved.

✓ Conversion rates from MCI to dementia are approximately 5-10% per year, while the yearly dementia incidence for cognitive normal individuals is 1-2%.

✓ Most people with MCI do not develop dementia.

✓ 25-50% of MCI cases revert to normal: their cognitive symptoms resolve.

✓ 37-67% of people diagnosed with MCI do not develop dementia or revert to normal but remain cognitively stable.

✓ A diagnosis of MCI should prompt a neurologic workup, but there is no treatment for MCI.

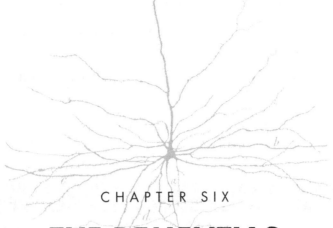

CHAPTER SIX
THE DEMENTIAS

It has been several years since Millie was diagnosed with Mild Cognitive Impairment, and she is now almost 84. Carol, her daughter, who is in her mid-50s, has monitored her mother's cognitive health with a cautious kind of optimism, hoping that her mother remains among the "stable" group of people with MCI—those who do not progress to dementia.

The first clues were subtle. Last spring, the garden, previously tidy, grew weeds, and the dahlias' unsupported stalks toppled in mid-summer under the weight of the flowers that Millie did not cut. She began to choose clothes that did not make sense for the weather or the social occasion. During happy hour, Millie participated less often in conversation. She now frequently starts a sentence but does not complete it, losing track of her idea or forgetting a critical word. She used to be a good cook, but now she seems to wander in the kitchen, forgetting her purpose or where to find the things she needs.

Carol knows that they must go back to the doctor.

Dementia is a condition of progressive cognitive decline that is abnormal for age, caused by a disease in the brain itself (rather than a problem with the thyroid or kidneys, for instance, or a medication or depression), and results in impairment of memory, mental processing, or judgement. Dementia symptoms may include not just forgetfulness, but changes in personality, mood, walking or other movements. "Dementia" is a general term. Within the general category of "dementia" are the specific dementias, each with its own name and characteristics.

95% of all people with dementia have one of the diagnoses explored in this chapter: Alzheimer's disease, vascular dementia, dementia with Lewy Bodies and the dementia associated with Parkinson's disease, frontotemporal dementia, and Normal Pressure Hydrocephalus.[1] The information in this chapter is not intended to be comprehensive. Rare dementias are not discussed because of the extremely low likelihood of relevance to the reader.[2] Detail has been heavily edited to give a general sense of each disease without overburdening the reader with particulars. The chapter is meant for those who are unfamiliar with the basic facts about dementia: dementia types, symptoms, evaluation, and treatment. For those who already have a good understanding of the subject—or perhaps those whose worry is easily exacerbated—it is a chapter than may be detoured.

---

[1] Gupta S, et al. Rare and Unusual Dementias. *Advances in psychiatric treatment* 2009;15: 364–371 DOI: 10.1192/apt.bp.107.003558

[2] For example, Creutzfeld-Jakob disease, Wilson disease, HIV-related dementia, dementias due to syphilis, or dementias secondary to diseases such as Huntington's disease, Multiple Systems Atrophy, Corticobasal syndrome, and variants of frontotemporal dementia and Parkinson's disease.

► Dementia is a condition of progressive cognitive decline.

► "Dementia" is a general diagnostic category, within which are dementias with specific names.

► The most common dementias, accounting for 95% of all dementia cases, are Alzheimer's dementia, vascular dementia, dementia with Lewy bodies/Parkinson's dementia, frontotemporal dementia, and normal pressure hydrocephalus.

► Each dementia has characteristic symptoms and findings on neurologic workup.

► *Read on to learn more*

1. ALZHEIMER'S DEMENTIA

"He was an attorney," his wife said, "But he can't work anymore. That's all over, his memory is terrible. He called me once when he got lost coming home. I tried to take away his car keys, but he hid them and then forgot where they were. I spent the whole morning looking for them. When I found the keys I didn't tell him, and the next day he'd forgotten the whole thing.

"I have to help him with his shirt buttons because otherwise he gets confused and buttons his shirt crooked, like a child. He leaves his clothes on the ground and wears them again the next day if I don't put them in the wash. We used to share the cooking, but now he can't follow a recipe or find a pan. I've always done the finances, which is a good thing because now he can't keep track of numbers. Like the time he tried to leave the house without socks. I told him to wear socks and he returned with three socks and an undershirt, holding them out like he wasn't sure what to do with them."

Alzheimer's dementia (AD) is the most common dementia after age 65, with 60-80% of all dementia cases in this age group due to AD.[3] 5-10% of all people over age 65 have AD, and after age 85 the prevalence increases to 30-50%. About 5% of Alzheimer's cases are "early onset," occurring prior to age 65. There is no cure for AD, and the medications available for treatment do not treat the disease but purport to boost cognition—though, inevitably, the

---

[3] *Alzheimers Dement* 2022;18(4):700-789. DOI: 10.1002/alz.12638

effect of the medications is minimal and temporary. AD is the 5th most common cause of death in people older than 65.[4]

Up close, brains with Alzheimer's disease typically show two abnormalities: "neurofibrillary tangles" and "beta amyloid plaques". These abnormalities are named for their appearance under the microscope: neurofibrillary tangles develop within neurons, filling them with abnormal protein, while beta amyloid plaques in an AD brain resemble many smeared black finger-prints—fuzzy, rounded, dark—within the brain but outside of the neurons themselves. (Beta amyloid plaques in AD are unrelated to other "plaques" that may develop in the body, such as plaques in arteries or on teeth.) Cognitive decline in AD correlates with increasing neurofibrillary tangles and amyloid plaques in the brain, particularly in the structures that support memory.

ALZHEIMER'S DISEASE: COGNITIVE FEATURES

While normal aging entails cognitive slowing and impairment of short-term memory, with relatively preserved longer-term memory and executive function, Alzheimer's disease is charac-terized by impairment in all these domains. The following table outlines the cognitive domains susceptible in AD.

---

[4] Arvanitakis Z, et al. Diagnosis and Management of Dementia: Review. *JAMA* 2019;322 (16). Gale SA, et al. Dementia. *The American Journal of Medicine* 2018; 131:1161–1169. DOI: 10.1016/j.amjmed.2018.01.022

COGNITIVE DOMAIN	EXAMPLES
Executive Function	**Normal abilities:** Planning, following through on tasks of multiple steps, multi-tasking, inhibition of disruptive or inappropriate impulses. **AD:** Difficulty with multi-step tasks (raking leaves then putting them in a bin, cleaning the kitchen, assembling a recipe), task incompletion, failure to pay bills, difficulty operating a car and navigating with a map, dressing properly for weather.
Episodic Memory	**Normal abilities:** Short-term memory tasks: where something was left, remembering a telephone number, address, flight number, or person's name. **AD:** Frequent misplacement of and keys and phone, forgetting appointments regularly, forgetting instructions entirely and immediately, needing to write down everything that cannot be forgotten.
Semantic Memory	**Normal abilities:** Language and skills acquired over a lifetime: using a telephone, spelling, mathematics, historical knowledge. **AD:** Limited vocabulary, loss of words that are not frequently used, inability to do math, frequent errors in spelling simple words, vagueness in discussing knowledge in which one was previously expert, helplessness with unfamiliar technology.
Language	**Normal abilities:** Understanding complex instructions, reading, writing, speaking fluently, naming, word recall. **AD:** Inability to follow verbal instructions, simplified vocabulary, empty and wandering sentences, misunderstanding simple instructions.

COGNITIVE DOMAIN	EXAMPLES
Visuospatial	**Normal abilities:** Drawing shapes, buttoning a shirt, making a bed, negotiating complex terrain, estimating the size and weight of an object. **AD:** Difficulty drawing simple shapes, confusion negotiating a park or neighborhood, confusion with stairs or escalators, inability to estimate the right amount of coffee grounds or condiment.
Behavioral	**Normal abilities:** Making socially appropriate conversation, interpreting verbal and non-verbal social cues, suppressing impulses that are rude, aggressive, or sexual. **AD:** Speaking out of turn in a conversation, making irrelevant comments, ignorance of emotions in others that are expressed non-verbally, making inappropriate sexual references.

Table 1: Cognitive Features of Alzheimer's Disease (AD)

The early stages of Alzheimer's disease are marked by trouble with recalling words and details, increasing in frequency such that the normal flow of daily activities is impaired. Conversation becomes characterized by repetitions, frequent word-searching, vagueness, side-stepping of complex ideas, increasingly short and fragmentary sentences. Longer sentences dead-end when the train of thought is lost or an important word forgotten. Impairment of other cognitive domains becomes evident with trouble using simple objects such as a telephone, remote control, scissors, or thermostat; care of the self and home is neglected; driving hazards emerge (getting lost or in accidents); and uncharacteristic oddness occurs in social interactions.

The compromise of multiple cognitive domains is the difference between AD and normal cognitive aging. In normal aging, there is slowing of cognitive speed and accuracy. It takes longer to remember something, and sometimes that thing just cannot be recalled at the moment it is needed. This is a problem with episodic memory. On the other hand, semantic memory is quite well preserved in normal aging: our fund of acquired learning is still available to us. Additionally, the cognitively normal middle-aged person's use and understanding of language is often better than a younger person's abilities. Also unaffected by normal aging is the ability to plan and follow through with tasks of multiple steps (for example, vacation planning: determining dates, buying airline tickets or planning the drive, renting a car or arranging transportation to a hotel, scheduling events, etc.). And there is no question but that the middle- or late-middle-aged possess an emotional maturity (often marked by patience, kindness, thoughtfulness, and selflessness) that is less consistently found in the young. Changes in just one of these domains, for instance, in episodic memory, is not incompatible with normal aging. But significant problems with several domains is a red flag for dementia.

ALZHEIMER'S DISEASE: EVALUATION

The evaluation of suspected Alzheimer's disease is twofold. First, other diseases must be ruled out (see Table 2, below, for more information). If no other cause of cognitive decline is found, then the second step in the workup seeks evidence supporting a diagnosis of AD.

PURPOSE	TEST

Rule out other causes of cognitive changes	• Blood tests:
	  • Thyroid, kidney, and liver function
	  • Vitamin B12 status
	  • If risk factors are present: HIV, syphilis, Lyme antibodies, heavy metals, autoimmune tests
	• Evaluate medication list
	• Query history of alcohol and drug abuse
	• Query history of psychiatric issues
	• Query history of insomnia
	• Brain MRI to evaluate for stroke, mass, autoimmunity, hydrocephalus

Evaluate for changes consistent with Alzheimer's disease	Brain MRI:
	  • Disproportionate hippocampal atrophy
	Neuropsychologic evaluation:
	  • Impairment in multiple cognitive domains (Executive function, memory, language, visuospatial, behavioral)
	Cerebrospinal fluid evaluation:
	  • High levels of tau, low levels of Aβ

Table 2: Dementia workup

In summary, the workup for AD is not complicated, but due diligence requires identifying any other cause of cognitive changes, and then proceeding with further testing, if needed, with brain imaging and/or neuropsychologic evaluation.

ALZHEIMER'S DISEASE: TREATMENT

There is no cure for Alzheimer's disease. Treatment is supportive, with caregivers eventually helping with cooking, transportation, shopping, management of finances, and basic self-care. In 2021 the FDA approved aducanumab for treatment of AD, but the data on which this approval was based was questionable, at best, and this medication will not significantly change the course of AD for most patients. There are some FDA-approved medications for cognitive support in AD.[5] While these medications help a minority of patients, the effects are not large and they are always temporary. The lack of effective treatment for AD makes the question of disease prevention particularly poignant.

2. VASCULAR DEMENTIA

"She has had a lot of medical problems for a long time," said her husband. "Heart attacks and strokes. She had blood clots in the legs. It was always hard for me to get her to take her blood pressure and diabetes meds, even before the dementia, because she would say that she didn't like meds and didn't like doctors. But now she won't take her medications at all unless I put the pills right in her hand. There's no way she would remember to take the pills herself.

"The forgetting started with her first stroke and then got worse with the second. And since the second stroke she has also had the weakness on the left side, so she has trouble doing almost anything for herself. Sometimes her I wonder if there have

---

[5] Donezepil, rivastigmine, and galantamine enhance the effects of acetylcholine in the brain, thereby augmenting cognitive function, while memantine works through inhibition of the NMDA receptors in the brain.

been other strokes, too, because her memory is getting worse and worse. There was a time when she seemed to be doing ok, her memory wasn't getting worse, but now…I've done my best with the meds but when we go to the doctor her blood sugar is still pretty high. I have to watch what she eats or when I check her sugar it's too high."

Vascular dementia is the second most common dementia and accounts for about 5-10% of all dementias.[6][7] Cognitive problems in vascular dementia are due to large or small strokes. Vascular dementia is suspected when, instead of a slow and regular progression of cognitive symptoms, abrupt worsening of cognition is followed by stability, followed by another episode of sudden decline. Risk factors are primarily cardiovascular, including high blood pressure, diabetes, high cholesterol, history of heart attack or other cardiac issues. Having vascular dementia may also increase the risk for dementia of other causes; the most common cause of "mixed dementia" is the combination of Alzheimer's and vascular dementias. Once vascular changes are visible on MRI, they cannot be resolved, but strict control of risk factors (normalization of blood pressure, blood glucose, and cholesterol) may slow progression of the disease.

---

[6] Some authors rank dementia with Lewy bodies as the second most common dementia after Alzheimer's dementia. In this case, they are ranking only the "neurodegenerative" dementias. Though usually progressive, vascular dementia is not considered strictly "neurodegenerative". Considering all dementias, however, vascular dementia is the second most common type.

[7] *Alzheimers Dement* 2022;18(4):700-789. DOI: 10.1002/alz.12638

3. DEMENTIA WITH LEWY BODIES, AND PARKINSON'S DISEASE DEMENTIA

"One day I just saw it. It had been there for months, the walking trouble, but somehow I hadn't noticed it," recalled his wife. "For some reason it was only when he was walking out of the restaurant that time that I really saw it, and then it was so obvious. The stooping and shuffling and the left arm that doesn't swing very much.

"Then he was diagnosed with Parkinson's disease and started taking medication and I realized that his memory had also been pretty bad. I realized that I had been reminding him about all kinds of things. Appointments, where we keep the coffee, the freeway exit. Now that he's on the medication he walks better and his memory isn't perfect but it's better than before. The odd thing is that he sometimes points out "little birds" in the house. The birds aren't really there, but when he first saw them I actually believed him. He was so sure about it. I don't know if it's a medication side effect or the Parkinson's itself. I don't say anything to the doctor because he is better on the medication and seeing the birds doesn't bother him. And on the meds, it's like I got some of him back."

Dementia with Lewy bodies (DLB) accounts for approximately 5% of all dementia diagnoses.[8] It is one of a handful of so-called "parkinsonian syndromes": conditions that are

---

[8] Gomperts SN. Lewy Body Dementias: Dementia With Lewy Bodies and Parkinson Disease Dementia. *Continuum* 2016;22(2):435–463

distinctly parkinsonian (slow movements, stooped and shuffling gait, increased tone in limbs) though different in key ways from Parkinson's disease. In dementia with Lewy bodies, cognitive symptoms present first, and movement abnormalities are less obvious. The cognitive changes are usually quite distinct, with visual hallucinations and fluctuations in level of consciousness (periods of prominent sleepiness; spells of good cognition followed by poor cognition) appearing early in the disease.

Dementia occurs in up to 78% of people with Parkinson's disease. Parkinson's disease symptoms, particularly earlier in the disease, are generally more obviously motor and less cognitive: resting tremor, slow movement, gait changes. Later, dementia may develop.

In the context of parkinsonism, cognitive symptoms such as visual hallucinations and spells of sleepiness or poor cognition indicate a likely diagnosis of dementia with Lewy bodies. Parkinson's disease dementia is more likely if the motor symptoms pre-date cognitive symptoms.

DLB and PDD: Evaluation

The workup of dementia in the context of parkinsonism is similar to the workup for Alzheimer's disease or vascular dementia. The evaluation should include blood testing, brain imaging, and neuropsychologic testing. (See Table 2, above.)

DLB and PDD: Treatment

As with many neurodegenerative diseases, the decline of function in dementia with Lewy bodies cannot be reversed, though a few medications may modestly improve symptoms. Some medications used for Alzheimer's disease can temporarily improve cognition in dementia with Lewy bodies and Parkinson's dementia. Because of the loss of the brain's dopamine-producing neurons is characteristic of both DLB and Parkinson's disease, supplementing with medications that enhance the activity of dopamine can improve cognitive symptoms in both diseases.

4. FRONTOTEMPORAL DEMENTIA

"They tell Mom that she has dementia but she doesn't believe it. Or maybe she doesn't even hear the doctor say it because she's thinking about the squirrels. It's another one of those things she's into these days. She talks about squirrels all the time. We had friends over, and Mom suddenly started talking about squirrels. Unrelated to the conversation. She's obsessed, even though she has zero contact with actual squirrels. She goes into the yard maybe once a month but then forgets why she's there. She comes back inside and right into my space, tapping my shoulder—hard, poking it—and drinking Chablis like it's water, which it actually is now because I pour out the wine and fill the bottle with apple juice and water.

"And it's not just the squirrels. She says odd things. I took her shopping and she told the check-out man that he looked heavy. She actually touched a mole on a stranger's face and said, 'What is that?' What do you say to apologize for something like that? Once, the whole family was going out to dinner and she came out the door wearing a bra and a green and white Portland Timbers scarf. And it wasn't a joke. I had to take her back in

*and get her dressed myself and she was angry about giving up
the scarf. She gets angry easily these days. Then, next thing,
she's embarrassingly touchy with the delivery person. And she
doesn't seem aware of the weirdness of any of it."*

Frontotemporal dementia (FTD) is the fourth most common
dementia after Alzheimer's disease, vascular dementia, and dementia
with Lewy bodies/Parkinson's dementia. After age 65, about 3%
of dementia cases are due to FTD.[9] There are several sub-types of
FTD, but the most common is the "behavioral variant," which is
the only FTD type discussed here. The behaviors caused by FTD
are bizarre, upsetting to family members, and difficult to treat.
Instead of a slow erasure of the outlines of the unique self—as with
Alzheimer's dementia or dementia with Lewy bodies—in frontotemporal dementia a new and obnoxious personality develops.
Later in the disease, the FTD patient's executive and motor disabilities outpace the behavioral issues, and language and walking
are severely limited. Soon thereafter the patient passes on, leaving
the family with memories of a difficult stranger.

Frontotemporal dementia, like Alzheimer's, can present before
age 65. Approximately 60% of all FTD cases occur between ages
40-64.[10] While executive dysfunction is a prominent aspect of
FTD, the most obvious problems are behavioral. In social situations, FTD patients are tactless, inappropriate, crude, and incon-
siderate. They joke excessively, make sexual remarks or advances,

[9] *Alzheimers Dement* 2022;18(4):700-789. DOI: 10.1002/alz.12638

[10] Bang J, et al. Non-Alzheimer's dementia 1: Frontotemporal dementia. *Lancet* 2015;386(10004): 1672–1682. DOI:10.1016/S0140-6736(15)00461-4

dress eccentrically, disregard personal space, urinate in public, and display no embarrassment or awareness otherwise that their behavior is abnormal. They are selfish and lack empathy. They may over-eat, preferring sweet to savory foods, drink alcohol excessively, gain weight, and become obsessed with certain words or phrases or ritualistic behaviors. They may impulsively over-spend, steal, gamble, or be involved in hit-and-run accidents. As the disease progresses, language and executive function decline severely, and death occurs 3-4 years after diagnosis.

Frontotemporal Dementia: Evaluation

The general workup of suspected frontotemporal dementia should again follow the steps indicated in Table 2. People with FTD may be mis-diagnosed with psychiatric disorders given the resemblance of some FTD behaviors to depression, obsessive-compulsive disorder, bipolar disorder, personality disorders, or schizophrenia. Making a diagnosis of FTD is aided by the distinct and unprecedented alteration in personality, and by the scope of the abnormal behaviors. Distinguishing FTD from psychiatric disorders becomes more straightforward as the condition progresses to involve domains of language and executive function.

10% of FTD cases have a strong family history of FTD, and 60% of these cases have genetic mutations. Testing for these gene mutations should be considered in patients with suspected FTD with a family history of dementia.

Frontotemporal Dementia: Treatment

As with the other degenerative dementias discussed— Alzheimer's disease, dementia with Lewy bodies—there is no cure for frontotemporal dementia. Treatment is aimed at behavioral management. Some medications used in AD and dementia with Lewy bodies can worsen FTD behaviors, and they have no role in treatment of FTD.

5. NORMAL PRESSURE HYDROCEPHALUS

"It started for me with the feet," he said. "I know that for some people it starts with the memory, or the bladder. But for me it started with the feet. They didn't respond to what my brain said. I could walk, but the feet were slow and heavy, and it was hard to get them off the ground. It was hard just to move forward. I fell a couple times. Within about six months, my memory was bad enough that I knew there was definitely something wrong. And then by the time I saw the neurologist I was actually losing control of my bladder. The whole thing...I felt kind of ashamed, like I was one of those helpless old people you see. I couldn't walk, couldn't remember anything. I wore adult diapers. But, a lot of the symptoms either disappeared or improved once I was treated. The tube is still in my brain, draining the fluid off, and I'm doing ok."

The final dementia to consider is normal pressure hydrocephalus (NPH). Unique among the dementias discussed in this chapter, NPH is fixable. It is caused by increased size of the ventricles (also called "hydrocephalus"). NPH involves a triad of symptoms: dementia, gait abnormalities, and urinary urgency and incontinence, though not all people with NPH have all three symptoms. The gait is typically described as "magnetic," with the feet scarcely lifting from the ground. Patients with dementia with Lewy bodies or Parkinson's disease dementia also shuffle, and this would seem to confuse the diagnosis, but NPH patients lack all other parkinsonian features such as tremor or slowness of movements.

Normal Pressure Hydrocephalus: Evaluation

Imaging is critical in establishing a diagnosis of NPH. A brain MRI or CT shows enlargement of the ventricles. If this is seen in the context of dementia and urinary incontinence, then NPH is possible.

Normal Pressure Hydrocephalus: Treatment

Treatment of NPH entails placing a tube, or shunt, in the ventricles. This allows the cerebrospinal fluid to drain and the brain to re-expand. The response of NPH to shunting depends, in part, to the duration of symptoms prior to treatment: the longer symptoms have been present, the less likely they will respond to treatment. Overall, the rate of subjective improvement after shunt placement is 96%, which is extremely high even considering the likelihood of a placebo effect. The chance of improvement walking speed is reported as 83%.[11]

Most people with dementia will have one of the dementias discussed here: Alzheimer's disease, vascular dementia, dementia with Lewy bodies/Parkinson's dementia, frontotemporal dementia, or

---

[11] Williams MA, Malm J. Diagnosis and Treatment of Idiopathic Normal Pressure Hydrocephalus. *Continuum* 2016;22(2):579-599

normal pressure hydrocephalus. Alzheimer's disease is the most common of all these dementias.

Carol's mother, Millie, had Mild Cogntive Impairment that was stable, but then her memory symptoms worsened. They returned to the doctor to re-evaluate her symptoms. Carol thought something was wrong, but she didn't know what her mother's diagnosis would be.

Carol and Millie: A Diagnosis

Memory testing at the doctor's office shows that Millie's cognition is worse than when it was tested several years ago. The doctor repeats the blood tests, again with normal results. A CT scan of Millie's brain shows "age-related changes" but no strokes, masses, or enlarged ventricles.

The doctor says that Millie probably has Alzheimer's disease, based on three facts. First, Millie's memory performance on testing is in the dementia range. Second, Millie has problems in multiple cognitive domains: episodic memory (forgetting things from moment-to-moment), language (word-finding difficulties), executive function and semantic memory (difficulty cooking and maintaining her garden) and behavior (choosing inappropriate clothes for social occasions). And third, blood tests and brain imaging do not indicate another cause for Millie's dementia. She doesn't have thyroid dysfunction, kidney problems, or stroke, and she has no other symptoms (walking trouble, urinary incontinence, tremor, personality changes) suggesting another kind of dementia.

The doctor gives Millie a prescription for a medication that may help boost her memory. But there is no cure for Alzheimer's, the doctor says. "What we need to focus on now is keeping your mother safe and maintaining her quality of life," says the doctor. "An important thing to consider first is whether you think she is safe to drive." Millie bristles at the idea that she may not be able to drive, insisting that there is nothing wrong. Carol drops it, for now.

There is a lot for Carol to think about. Her mother's wellbeing is important to her, and she wants to do a good job taking care of her. Carol has so many questions, and the first one out of her mouth is, "Will she be unhappy?" The second question— the one she doesn't ask aloud—is: "Does this mean that I will get dementia, too?"

It is not just the cognitive impairment that makes dementia menacing to those who worry but also the decline. Watching a family member's deterioration—as Carol must watch her mother's—raises the question of one's own risk for dementia. When Millie was forgetful but did not have dementia—when she had Mild Cognitive Impairment—Carol felt reassured that genetics were on her side, that at least her own risk for dementia was not increased by a family history of the disease. But now that her mother has Alzheimer's disease, Carol's concern for her own brain revives. She needs information. She needs clear answers about her own dementia risk. Is dementia genetic? How much, exactly, does a mother with dementia increases Carol's own dementia risk? What are the numbers? In the next chapter, we will learn what a family history of dementia means for Carol, and for you.

🔔 REMEMBER:

✓ Dementia is a condition of progressive cognitive decline that is abnormal for age and results in impairment of memory, mental processing, and/ or judgement.

✓ "Dementia" is a general diagnostic category, within which are dementias with specific names.

✓ The most common dementias, accounting for 95% of all dementia cases, are Alzheimer's dementia, vascular dementia, dementia with Lewy bodies/ Parkinson's dementia, frontotemporal dementia, and normal pressure hydrocephalus.

✓ Each dementia has characteristic symptoms and findings on neurologic workup.

✓ Except for normal pressure hydrocephalus, these dementias cannot be cured.

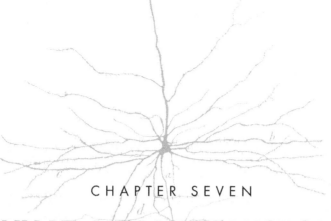

CHAPTER SEVEN

WHAT A FAMILY HISTORY
OF ALZHEIMER'S DEMENTIA
MEANS FOR YOU

"Alzheimer's disease runs in my family."
This seems like a straightforward reporting of fact.
Someone in the family had Alzheimer's disease (AD).

And perhaps that relative shared certain other characteristics
with other family members: a nose, a way of speaking, wavy hair,
an aptitude for math, or a body shape. Or perhaps the affected
family member was particularly close with her great niece, and
there is a family understanding that the two are deeply similar in
a way that is as good as genetic, putting the great niece at special
risk for AD.

With this understanding of heritability, it is natural to worry
that having a family member with Alzheimer's disease increases
the AD risk for the whole family. Genetics do influence the risk
for Alzheimer's disease, but not usually in such broad way within
a family. The more that is known about an individual's genetic

history, the more precise can be the determination of an individual's AD risk.

- ▶ For many people with a family history of AD, their true risk for AD is different than their perceived risk.

- ▶ Genes can influence risk for AD, and a family history of the disease may increase an individual's lifetime risk for the disease.

- ▶ Other genetic factors that influence an individual's lifetime risk for AD are gender, ethnicity, and *APOE* genotype.

- ▶ *Read on to learn more.*

1. DREAD AND FAMILIARITY

Worry flourishes in ignorance. Like a weed in a sidewalk crack, worry can germinate from almost nothing: information that is incomplete, decontextualized, or unreliable. Health worries feed on an anecdotal Facebook story, the experience of an acquaintance's cousin, or an unlucky landing on an ominous internet page; and, in this way, they resemble tomato plants cultivated upside down, their roots implausibly in air, tomatoes dangling below—yet they thrive.

Worry is risk transformed by the prism of emotion. It is not always an inaccurate detector of risk, though it often distorts or exaggerates the degree of actual risk, like the warped world that appears when a prism is held to the eye. If one has the tendency to look for it, risk is everywhere, as suggested in the following list of "activities and technologies" shown to participants in a study of how people perceive risk:[1]

Nuclear power	Spray cans
Electric power	Bicycles
Motor vehicles	Contraception
Swimming	Skiing
Handguns	X-rays
Smoking	Railroads
Alcoholic beverages	Food preservatives
Pesticides	Power mowers
Surgery	Food coloring
Hunting	Home appliances

---

[1] Paul Slovic, et al. *Facts and Fears: Societal Perception of Risk*, in NA - Advances in Consumer Research Volume 08, eds. Kent B. Monroe, Ann Abor, MI. 1981

All these activities or technologies entail some risk, though some are riskier (motor vehicles, smoking) than others (home appliances). Some are obviously worth worrying about (guns), some are not (spray cans), and the risk associated with some technologies, such as nuclear power or alcoholic beverages, depends on the perspective from which you choose to view them. Many of the participants of this study ranked nuclear power as the riskiest, yet actuaries know that the most dangerous of these activities, by far, is driving a car. In these participants' responses we see that there is something more at play in people's understanding of risk than risk itself. Calculated risk and beliefs about risk are not the same thing; the actual amount of risk entailed by an activity or technology and the amount of worry generated by it are not necessarily the same.

When we speak of beliefs about risk and their connection to actual risk, we are speaking of a concept called "perception of personal risk". Perception of personal risk is not determined by math, alone; there is an emotional component that drives the relevance of the risk for the individual. For those who worry that they might develop dementia, their concern is probably based less often on an accurate understanding of their true risk and more often on fears generated by vivid examples of dementia in their personal life, movies, or internet jive. My worry that I had Alzheimer's disease as a twenty-year-old—and my perception of risk—contained almost no factual element and was entirely driven by a fear that appeared, not coincidentally, at the same time that I was challenged by a college curriculum.

The point is that, for the individual, the significance of a family history of dementia is twofold: one aspect is emotional (the fear of dementia is embodied by a relative afflicted with the disease), the other medical (the genetics that may or may not be shared in a family). The two get mixed up—the powerful emotional consequences of first-hand experience with the disease strengthens one's perception of personal risk for the disease. And in the absence of data on which to ground oneself, worry has free rein to dictate perception of risk.

Few medical problems have more potential to create worry than does dementia. Perhaps only cancer has a similar power. Both conditions are "seen as involuntary, delayed, unknown, uncontrollable, unfamiliar, potentially catastrophic, dreaded, and severe"— the characteristics that most readily elicited dread for the participants in the study of risk discussed above. Thus, the study participants' high risk rating for nuclear power: though harm due to nuclear technology is exceedingly rare, cases of nuclear catastrophe, such as Chernobyl or Three Mile Island, are vivid in our minds. Risks that we cannot control, that we do not understand, and that are catastrophic are perceived as more threatening and more dreaded than risks that, however common, are avoidable, familiar, and less catastrophic, such as x-rays. The axes of worry are dread and familiarity: perception of personal risk increases with dread, but it diminishes as the object of worry is better understood.

With these ideas in mind, it makes sense that dread may be reduced by shifting one's understanding of personal risk as close as possible to actual risk. In the case of dementia, this would mean developing a more realistic understanding of one's lifetime risk for developing the disease. But there are barriers to acquiring this information. While many resources are available for the patient with dementia there is little organized information for the lay person concerned about their personal risk for dementia. Another barrier to information acquisition is emotional: watching a family member's cognitive decline discourages frank contemplation of one's own risk. Yet if we do not directly confront our own risk for dementia the mind will do it indirectly, weirdly, the imagination distorting risk in the absence of factual guidance. Our minds, grappling with the fear of a disease that is involuntary, delayed, uncontrollable, catastrophic, and severe, grow tomatoes of dread upside down, the roots of worry feeding on nothing more solid than air.

This is also Carol's experience. Her mother's diagnosis of Alzheimer's disease reawakens her concern that she, too, could develop dementia. Concern becomes worry, and her worry, unrestrained by facts, begins to grow.

Carol and Millie: Family

Carol is spinning. She is sure she is going to be demented, just like her mother. She has no control over the situation—how can she change her genes?—and this increases her anxiety. Who will take care of her? She is unmarried and without children. Her brother lives on the other side of the country and has his own family. Carol sees her future self alone in a care facility. And care facilities are expensive. Does she have enough money saved? How many more years will she be able to work?

Carol's nose has become ominous to her. She has always liked her nose. It's attractive, she thinks, and it's exactly like her mother's. She admires her mother and likes that they share a nose. But now her nose has a different significance. Seeing her mother and looking in the mirror at herself, her nose reminds her of the genes she shares with her mother. If they share a nose, then they must share dementia genes.

For the first time ever, her connection to her mother isn't a source of pride but of worry. Her brother looks more like their father, so she guesses he would have mostly their father's genes. Their father passed from cancer ten years ago, and there's no telling whether he would have developed dementia, but her brother probably has a lower dementia risk than Carol.

Carol's worry grows until one day it overwhelms her. She calls a friend, who eventually asks her a question that is outlandish but thoughtful: If you were at work, and a client wanted to invest not in a company but in you—Carol—what would you recommend? The client wants a good investment in someone who will be healthy and productive for a long time. "How would you advise the client?" asks her friend. "Are you going to be healthy and productive for a long time? Do you think you have enough information to advise the client at all, one way or the other?" This perspective is different than Carol's gut-level approach to dementia. "You can't just shoot from the hip," her friend reminds her. "You have to know the numbers to understand your future."

Carol remembers the conversation with her friend as a revelation. The knot inside her chest loosens. Her friend is right:

Carol doesn't really know the numbers. She doesn't know her actual risk for dementia. She is startled that she never thought of her situation in this way before, using facts. Her worry for dementia was based on imagination and intuition—poor tools for building an investment strategy for a client, and poor tools for building an understanding of her dementia risk.

Carol acknowledges that she doesn't really know very much about genetics. She also sees that for her a better understanding of the true risk for dementia will go a long way in managing her worry.

Carol cannot change her family history of dementia. But dread can be eased by illuminating the actual, calculated risk in the context of a family history of the disease. If Carol gains a better understanding of her true dementia risk, her worry for dementia may diminish. Numbers do not often give answers that are completely free of ambiguity, but do they give answers that are honest and accurate. In the next section, we will consider the risk for Alzheimer's disease for all people. Then we will examine risk in the context of a family history of the disease. Finally, we will explore genetic aspects of early-onset and late-onset Alzheimer's disease, and we will learn how AD risk is influenced by age, gender, ethnicity, and the *APOE* gene.

2. ALZHEIMER'S DISEASE GENETICS

Understanding the hereditary aspects of Alzheimer's disease requires a working knowledge of a few important genetic concepts. In the nucleus of most human cells are chromosomes. Each chromosome is a collection of DNA unique to each individual (except in the case of identical twins). Within each strand of DNA are many thousands of regions, or genes. The language of a gene is translated by the cell into a protein that serves a specific function in the body. The genes within DNA, therefore, are the source for all the elements necessary for the normal functioning of the body.

Some DNA regions are unexpressed, or silent. They are not translated and they produce no effect on the body. Other regions of DNA contain genes that are always expressed, and these are called "deterministic" genes. If one possesses a deterministic gene for a disease, there is a 100% chance of developing that disease. Other genes—so-called "susceptibility genes"— have a less than 100% chance of being expressed. Susceptibility genes increase risk for a disease but the risk is not 100%. In the next few paragraphs we will see that deterministic genes and susceptibility genes play an important role in the genetics of Alzheimer's disease.

The discovery of deterministic genes for Alzheimer's disease was the key to researchers' initial understanding of the causes of the disease and to the development of the "Amyloid Hypothesis." In 1907, Alois Alzheimer described a 53-year-old patient with brain abnormalities that were later called plaques and neurofibrillary tangles—findings seen under the microscope in brains of people with AD. The content of AD-related brain plaques remained mysterious for decades, until in the 1980s the substance was found to be Beta amyloid, often called "β-amyloid."

To understand the role of β-amyloid in Alzheimer's disease, researchers had to understand how it was made. A clue to the source of β-amyloid was afforded by Down's syndrome. The prevalence of Alzheimer's disease in the Down's syndrome population is almost 100% after age 60. It was suggested that the cause for this high prevalence was related to the genetic abnormality carried by all people with Down's syndrome: they have three copies of chromosome 21 instead of the usual two copies, which abnormally increases production of the protein, which in turn causes Alzheimer disease pathology to develop so easily in Down's syndrome brains. In people with or without Down's syndrome, excessive brain β-amyloid triggers a host of responses in neurons and other brain cells that result in brain damage and the clinical symptoms of Alzheimer's disease.

In the 1990s, the first deterministic genes for AD were identified in families with a strong history of AD that presented early in life. In these families with Early Onset Alzheimer's Disease (EOAD), anyone with the gene was almost certain to develop AD before age 65. Thus far, three such genes have been identified. Two of them are fully deterministic (100% of people with a gene will get AD), and one of the genes is almost fully deterministic, with 95% of people with the gene developing AD.

Fortunately, less than 2% of all cases of Alzheimer's disease are early onset. Most AD is diagnosed after age 65 and called Late Onset Alzheimer's Disease, or LOAD, and most LOAD is not caused by deterministic genes. In fact, when we talk about the genetics of late onset AD (which is over 98% of all cases of Alzheimer's disease) we are mainly talking about susceptibility genes: genes that increase risk for AD but do not guarantee that the disease will develop. This is an important point to acknowledge: most genes that increase risk for AD do not guarantee it, and plenty of people with a family of history of Alzheimer's disease will not get it themselves. Practically speaking, there is only one relevant susceptibility gene for AD: the Apolipoprotein E (*APOE*) gene.

The discovery of the *APOE* gene and the protein that it encodes for, APOE, gave researchers a crucial tool for understanding Alzheimer's disease.[2] Many scientific papers have been published about *APOE* and the effects of the APOE protein on the brain, exploring how the APOE protein facilitates and even directly causes damage to brain cells in AD. To know the effects of the *APOE* on the brain is to understand much about the causes of Alzheimer's disease.

APOE genetics at first seem a little complicated, but they are not so difficult to understand, and a good grasp of them will be useful in understand dementia risk. In brief, every individual has two copies of the *APOE* gene, and each gene copy comes in one of three possible varieties, or alleles:[3] *APOE2*, *APOE3*, and *APOE4*. (The names for these alleles can be abbreviated E2, E3, and E4.)

The most common *APOE* gene is E3, followed by E4, then E2.[4] Whether E2, E3, or E4, the APOE protein serves an import-

---

[2] By convention, a gene is italicized ("*APOE*"), while the protein produced by the gene is not ("APOE").

[3] Alleles are varieties of a single gene. If there were a single gene that determined human hair color, for example, one allele of this gene would code for brown hair, another allele would code for black hair, another allele for red hair, etc.

[4] One study showed the following frequencies of *APOE* gene types among a large group of older people. Any E3 (eg, E3/E3, E3/E4, or E3/E2): 92.8%. Any E4: 32.3%. Any E2: 16.5%. Also: E3/3 54.1%, E3/4 25.8%, E4/E4 2.9%. Breitner JCS, *et al. APOE*-E4 count predicts age when prevalence of AD increases, then declines: The Cache County Study. *Neurology* 1999;53:321–331

ant cellular function: the APOE protein picks up fats and transports them from brain cell to cell for use in cell repair and maintenance. Fats are particularly important in brain tissue, which contains a high percentage of fat. Each APOE protein type binds fats differently, with APOE4 binding them more poorly than APOE3, which binds them more poorly than APOE2. This fact is relevant because risk for Alzheimer's disease follows the same order: dementia risk is greatest with the E4 allele, followed by E3, then E2. We will consider these risks in more detail presently.[5]

The research gives a clear picture of *APOE*'s influence on Alzheimer's disease risk. Multiple studies of large numbers of patients come to the same conclusions. The E2 allele is protective against dementia (people with the E2 gene are less likely than people with E3 or E4 to get dementia). The E3 allele neither increases nor reduces risk for Alzheimer's disease (it is "neutral"). And the E4 allele increases dementia risk.

It is important to state clearly, again, that the *APOE4* gene is a susceptibility gene: having it does not ensure dementia. There are cognitively normal people who carry two *APOE4* genes, just as there are AD patients who do not have the E4 gene.

---

[5] There is more to APOE and Alzheimer's risk than just differences in lipid binding. APOE4—but not APOE3 or APOE2—may also directly cause AD changes in the brain through a variety of other mechanisms, many of them related to APOE4 and β-amyloid interactions. APOE4 may increase β-amyloid collection in the brain, inefficiently clear it from the brain, or alter its shape to promote deposition in the brain. APOE4 may inefficiently remove free radicals from the brain, and it may promote inflammation or be directly neurotoxic.

3. FAMILIAL/GENETIC FACTORS AND RISK FOR AD

Having reviewed Alzheimer's disease genetics, we now come to this chapter's purpose: to answer the reader's concern for AD in the context of a family history of the disease. It is important to point out that studies examining risk in families of people with Alzheimer's disease focus on a specific family situation: the risk of dementia for first-degree relatives of people with dementia. A "first-degree relative" means a parent, sibling, or child. As a result, a discussion of dementia risk in families only applies to people with a parent, sibling, or child with dementia. We do not have much information about other family history scenarios—say, an uncle or cousin or grandparent with dementia (so-called "second-degree" relatives). That is not to say that dementia risk is not influenced by a second-degree relative—we just do not have the data to prove this is so or what the risk might be.

There are a lot of numbers in the following sections, and not all of numbers are relevant to every reader. In fact, much of the chapter will not apply to most readers, whose gender and ethnic identifications will differ. Unless you have a general interest in the subject of AD and its genetic influences, I suggest scanning the section headings and reading only those that apply to you. Consider also looking over "Table A: Genetic/Familial Factors and Risk for Alzheimer's Disease," which summarizes AD risk and is included at the end of the book.

The background risk for AD is about 10-12%. If nothing is known about an individual's personal health history or family history, the risk of developing AD over a lifetime is 10-12%. (A "lifetime" is usually assumed to be 80-85 years.) Another way to understand this estimate is to consider yourself and nine of your friends: the odds are that one of you will have AD by age 85. To calibrate your sense of risk, consider that a 10-12% lifetime risk for AD is lower than the lifetime risk of dying of any kind of cancer, which is about 20%.[6]

We will see that an individual's risk for Alzheimer's disease changes, for better or worse, depending on how much we know about the individual, and that from this background lifetime risk for AD of 10-12% we can further refine AD risk estimates by accounting for age, gender, ethnicity, and *APOE* genotype.

The background risk for Alzheimer's disease varies with age. The prevalence of dementia before age 65 is probably less than 1%. After age 65 the prevalence increases. Among those age 65-74, the AD prevalence is 5.3%. From ages 75-84 the prevalence is 13.8%, and after age 85 the prevalence is 34.6%.[7] Stated another way, increasing age is the strongest risk factor for AD because, unlike genetic variables that differ among individuals, aging is an exposure equally suffered by all.

Background risk for Alzheimer's varies with gender. Most studies show that women are more likely to get AD than men. The conclusions of one very large study are probably representative of the overall findings in the literature: the lifetime risk for AD is about

[6] https://www.cancer.org/cancer/cancer-basics/lifetime-probability-of-developing-or-dying-from-cancer.html

[7] Kumar B. Rajan, KB, et al. Population estimate of people with clinical Alzheimer's disease and mild cognitive impairment in the United States (2020–2060). *Alzheimer's Dement.* 2021;1–10. DOI: 10.1002/alz.1236

twice as high in women as in men.[8] In this study, the lifetime risk for AD was 20% for women and 10% for men. This study, and others, put a still finer point on gender and risk for AD: women's risk for AD relative to men probably emerges only after about age 75-80, as demonstrated in the following graph.

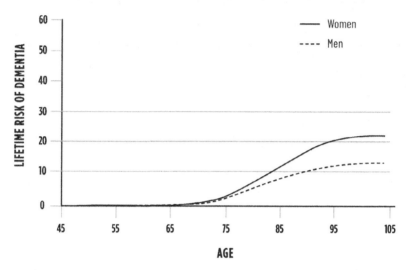

Figure 1: Women have a higher risk for Alzheimer's disease than men in late life

(Adapted from: Chene, G, et al. Gender and incidence of dementia in the Framingham Heart Study from mid-adult life. Alzheimers Dement. 2015 March ; 11(3): 310–320.)

On this graph, the risk of AD for men and women tracks upwards together beginning at age 65 until about age 75-80, at which time the risk for women increases relative to men. This effect may be due to the increased likelihood of men dying at an earlier age from stroke or heart attack. Cardiovascular disease can

---

[8]   Chene, G, et al. Gender and incidence of dementia in the Framingham Heart Study from mid-adult life. *Alzheimers Dement.* 2015 March ; 11(3): 310–320. doi:10.1016/j.jalz.2013.10.005

augment the degenerative changes of dementia, and males who do not die of heart attack or stroke may, as a group, have less cardiovascular disease, may be more cognitively fit, and may therefore be less likely to develop AD.

The background risk for AD varies with ethnicity. (Please see footnote[9] for a comment on nomenclature.) The prevalence of dementia varies with ethnicity, affecting 10% of Whites, 14% of Hispanics, and 18% of African Americans after age 65. Less information is available regarding AD risk among other ethnicities, but large studies have shown an AD prevalence of 10.5% for Native Americans, 10.1% for Asian and Pacific Islanders, and 6.3% among Japanese subjects.

---

[9] This book endorses the following opinion on use of "race" versus "ethnicity" from Kurt Christensen (Christensen KD, et al. Incorporating ethnicity into genetic risk assessment for Alzheimer disease: the REVEAL study experience. *Genet Med.* 2008:10(3):207–214): "Although the terms 'race' and 'racial' occasionally appear in this article, this does not mean that the authors subscribe to the view that the human species sub-structures into biological races. The terms are being used because of their presence in the relevant literature. 'Ethnicity' and 'ethnic' are our preferred (and dominant) terms, as we believe that they more accurately describe the primary groups on which our study focuses." Additionally, with full acknowledgement of the complexities of ethnic identification and the inadequacy of any single method to accommodate the naming preferences of all people in all groups, as well as the limited diversity of ethnicities actually studied by the scientific literature, for pragmatic purposes this book will resort to the unfortunately simplified nomenclature used by the US Census when referring to the larger ethnic groupings of "African American", "Hispanic", "White", "Asian and Pacific Islander", and "American Indian and Alaskan Native".

The following is a graph of AD prevalence for each US Census ethnic category.[10] An AD percentage of 13.8 for African American males means that, within a group confined only to African American males 65 or older, 13.8% have AD. (This is approximately, but not exactly, the same as lifetime risk for AD.)

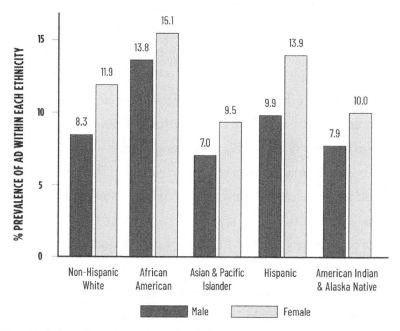

Figure 2: Estimated prevalence of Alzheimer's disease by gender and US Census categories

(Adapted from: Matthews, KA, et al. Racial and ethnic estimates of Alzheimer's disease and related dementias in the United States (2015–2060) in adults aged ≥65 years. Alzheimers Dement. 2019 January ; 15(1): 17–24.)

Averaging the risk for men and women within each group on this graph, Asian & Pacific Islanders have the lowest AD risk

---

[10] Matthews, KA, et al. Racial and ethnic estimates of Alzheimer's disease and related dementias in the United States (2015–2060) in adults aged ≥65 years. *Alzheimers Dement.* 2019 January ; 15(1): 17–24. doi:10.1016/j.jalz.2018.06.3063

in this study (8.25%), followed by American Indian & Alaska Natives (8.95%), followed by Non-Hispanic Whites (10.1%), and Hispanics (11.9%). In this study, African Americans have the highest risk for AD at 14.45%. (Note also that this graph confirms the increased prevalence of dementia in females compared to males within all ethnicities.)

Having surveyed estimates of risk for AD by ethnicity, it is a good idea to step back and question the generalizability and reliability of data based on ethnicity. There are multiple objections to using ethnicity in scientific studies and just a few of them are noted here. First, investigations of non-White ethnicities often use samples too small to generate much statistical power—such small studies are not reliable and their conclusions should not be accepted until replicated by larger studies. Second, ethnic self-identification may be a poor proxy for genetic risk. Ethnicity is often a cultural and not a genetic identification, and self-reporting of ethnicity does not necessarily correspond to actual genetic background (as discovered by many who are surprised by their 23andMe results). Third, there is much genetic diversity within ethnic categories. For example, the U.S. Census category, "Asian and Pacific Islander," encompasses Chinese, Filipinos, Vietnamese, Koreans, Hawaiians, Indonesians, and others—to say nothing of the myriad more specific ethnicities within each of these broader categories. Other ethnic categories can be similarly atomized: "White" could mean Russian, Swiss, Spanish, Greek, Lebanese; "African" in "African American" might encompass any genetic background from Egyptian to Namibian; "Hispanic" could indicate, among other affiliations, such potentially dissimilar genetic backgrounds as Spanish or Mexican.

Finally, ethnic identifications entail cultural, psychological, and socioeconomic realities that affect AD risk in ways that are non-genetic. For instance, consider an ethnic identification associated with dietary practices that increase cardiovascular disease risk that can, in turn, increases risk for dementia. Consider also how the wider cultural landscape can influence disease in an ethnic subgroup, as described by Kurt Christensen, et al[11]: "Health disparities are typically the result of many factors, including socioeconomic inequalities, social environment, health care access, health behaviors, and discrimination, and it is likely that at least some of these factors contribute to the disproportionate burden of AD." It is unsound to conclude that an ethnicity's higher dementia rate is due to a genetic tendency, alone, when instead a multitude of non-genetic factors may be at play. One study of AD and ethnicity expressed skepticism that useful conclusions may be drawn regarding variable AD risk among ethnic categories as currently characterized, concluding that, "We cannot comment on any biological differences which may account for differences in incidence [of AD]," and further stating that "Disaggregation of large race/ethnic classifications is warranted due to within-population heterogeneity"—that is, ethnic groups may contain an overlooked diversity of genetic content, and studies that ignore this diversity are liable to draw mistaken conclusions.[12] Studies of ethnicity and risk are more reliable when their scope is confined to a relatively

---

[11] Christensen KD, et al. Incorporating ethnicity into genetic risk assessment for Alzheimer disease: the REVEAL study experience. *Genet Med* 2008:10(3):207–214

[12] Mehta KM, et al. Systematic review of dementia prevalence and incidence in United States race/ethnic populations. *Alzheimers Dement.* 2017;72-83

homogeneous and genetically stable population. For example, it would be better to focus a study of the genetic underpinnings of AD on the more limited category of "Mexicans" rather than the broader group of "Hispanics," and it would be better still to study not "Mexicans" but "Yucatan Mayans."

This is not to say that we should not study health conditions and their potential associations with ethnicity. In fact, it is critical to investigate the patterns of disease in diverse populations. This is obvious. The point is that, when searching for genetic causes of disease, ethnic identification may be misleading because it is a poor proxy for genetics.

Alzheimer's disease risk differs for families with a history of early onset versus late onset AD. Two paths, each with different risks, diverge from a first-degree family history of AD. (Recall that a "first-degree relative" is a parent, sibling, or child.) The first path begins with a family history of early-onset AD (EOAD). In this case, the family may carry one of the genes that ensures onset of AD symptoms before age 65. Remember that early-onset Alzheimer's disease accounts for less than 2% of all AD cases. EOAD is rare, and most people with a concern for developing AD will not find themselves in this group.

The second and much more common risk pathway begins with a first-degree family member with late onset AD (LOAD). In late onset AD, dementia is not inevitable for family members, but risk is increased. The following discussion is confined to late onset AD, because LOAD accounts for about 98% of all AD.

By age 96, the cumulative lifetime risk of AD for anyone with a first-degree family history of AD is 39%, according to one large study.[13] In this study, males had a 30.9% lifetime risk for AD, while females had a 43.9% risk. Three other studies demonstrate similar findings, with a range of Alzheimer's disease among 1st-degree relatives of AD patients of 40-46%.[14] Recall that the background AD lifetime risk—the risk for AD if nothing is known about gender, ethnicity, family history, or *APOE* genotype—is about 10-12%. A positive 1st-degree family history of AD is a powerful AD risk factor—though by no means does it ensure that AD will develop.

The APOE4 gene increases Alzheimer's disease risk. Here the statistics begin to get weedy. This is unfortunately inevitable; the language of medical science is often spoken in statistics, which is comfortable for statisticians but difficult for the rest of us. We will press on because the information is important to anyone who wishes to fine-tune their sense of Alzheimer's disease risk.

As noted already, every individual has two copies of the *APOE* gene, one from each parent. Each gene copy comes in one of three possible variants, or alleles[15]—E2, E3, or E4—each resulting in a

---

[13] Lautenschlager NT, et al. Risk of dementia among relatives of patients in the MIRAGE study: What is in store for the oldest old? *Neurology.* 1996;46:641-650

[14] Farrer LA, et al. Apolipoprotein E Genotype in Patients with Alzheimer's Disease: Implications for the Risk of Dementia Among Relatives. *Ann Neurol.* 1995;38:797-808, Martinez M, et al. Apolipoprotein E e4 Allele and Familial Aggregation of Alzheimer Disease. *Arch Neurol.* 1998;55:810-816, Green RC, et al. Risk of Dementia Among White and African American Relatives of Patients With Alzheimer Disease. *JAMA.* 2002;287:329-336

[15] Alleles are varieties of a single gene. If there were a single gene that determines human hair color, for example, one allele of this gene codes for brown hair, another allele codes for black hair, another allele for red hair, etc..

unique risk for AD. The E2 allele is considered protective against AD, while the E3 allele is neutral, neither increasing nor decreasing AD risk above the background risk. The E4 gene increases risk for AD in an additive way: a single E4 copy increases risk by a factor of about 3-4, and two copies of the E4 gene increases risk for AD by a factor of about 8.

The following graph illustrates the increased AD risk posed by having one or two copies of the E4 gene compared with having the E2 and/or E3 gene:[16]

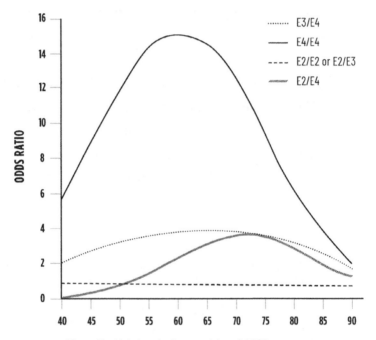

Figure 3: Alzheimer's disease risk and APOE genotype

(Adapted from: Farrer LA, et al. Effects of age, sex, and ethnicity on the Association Between Apolipoprotein E Genotype and Alzheimer Disease. JAMA. 1997:278:1349-1356)

---

[16] Farrer LA, et al. Effects of age, sex, and ethnicity on the Association Between Apolipoprotein E Genotype and Alzheimer Disease. *JAMA.* 1997:278:1349-1356

Here the risk for AD is expressed on the vertical axis as an odds ratio (OR).[17] The higher the odds ratio, the higher the risk for AD. There is an obvious difference in risk for AD in subjects with one E4 gene compared with E2 or E3 carriers, with the E4 carriers having about three times the AD risk. There is a still greater and more visually dramatic difference between the risk curve for a single E4 allele (odds ratio of about 3) compared with the risk with two E4 alleles (odds ratio about 14), demonstrating again the "*APOE*4 dose effect": the greater the E4 dose (the more copies of the allele possessed by an individual), the greater the risk for AD.

APOE4's effect on AD risk is age-dependent. Not only does APOE4 increase the risk for AD, but it shifts the onset of symptoms to a younger age. Individuals with AD and the APOE4 gene are likely to be younger when they develop symptoms than those who do not possess the APOE4 gene. The average age of onset of AD in individuals without the E4 gene is about age 80-85. Having one E4 gene reduces the average age of onset of AD to about age 75, while two E4 genes bring the average age of AD onset to 70. One study concluded that for each copy of the E4 gene the average age of onset of AD symptoms is reduced by eight years.[18]

---

[17] An odds ratio (OR) compares the likelihood of an event (for example, developing Alzheimer's disease) occurring in one group (for example, people with the E4 gene) compared to another group (people with the E3 gene). An OR of 2 means that a group has double the risk of an event compared with another group. In this study, the group of people with the E3/E3 genotype were assumed to have a "neutral" AD risk (neither increased nor decreased), and the AD risk for other groups were compared against the E3/E3 group.

[18] Mahley R. Apolipoprotein E: from cardiovascular disease to neurodegenerative disorders. *J Mol Med.* 2016; 94:739–746 DOI 10.1007/s00109-016-1427-y

The age-dependency of the E4 effect is illustrated by the following graph, which we saw already in our discussion of the over-all increased risk for AD posed by the *APOE*4 gene.[19]

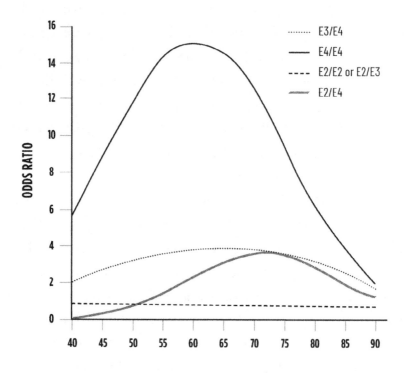

Figure 3: Alzheimer's disease risk and APOE genotype

(Adapted from: Farrer LA, et al. Effects of age, sex, and ethnicity on the Association Between Apolipoprotein E Genotype and Alzheimer Disease. JAMA. 1997:278:1349-1356)

On this graph, the peak AD risk for the E3/4 genotype is at about age 65. The E4/E4 genotype peaks earlier, at about age 60. We see, then, that the E4 dose effect is twofold: two copies of the

---

[19] Farrer LA, et al. Effects of age, sex, and ethnicity on the Association Between Apolipoprotein E Genotype and Alzheimer Disease: a Meta-analysis. *JAMA.* 1997:278:1349-1356

E4 gene increase AD lifetime risk more than does a single copy of the gene; and the greater the E4 dose, the earlier the onset of AD symptoms.[20]

The APOE4 gene influences AD risk for all ethnicities. Most studies of the APOE4 gene enlist White subjects and include few participants of other ethnicities. It is fair to ask what this literature can offer non-White ethnicities wishing to understand their risk for AD. Can we assume that if the APOE4 gene increases risk in Whites it does so in other ethnicities?

Studies do confirm an increased *APOE4*-associated AD risk among most ethnicities.[21] The general consistency of the *APOE4* effect over many ethnicities suggests that while it may not be possible to include large numbers of every ethnicity in every study, it is at least plausible that most studies' conclusions are applicable to most people.

African Americans: With one E4 gene, the risk for an African American individual of developing AD is increased by a factor of 2.0-2.6. Having two E4 genes increases the risk by a factor of 7.0-10.5. After Whites, there are more studies on the *APOE* effect among African-Americans than any other ethnic group.

---

[20] The E2/E4 genotype's risk peaks in this graph at age 70. Recall that the E2 gene is protective against AD; pairing it with an E4 gene probably partially offsets the increased risk posed by the E4 gene.

[21] Yorubans and Amish are exceptions. See: Murrell JR, et al. Association of Apolipoprotein E Genotype and Alzheimer Disease in African Americans. *Arch Neurol.* 2006 March ; 63(3): 431–434. DOI:10.1001/archneur.63.3.431

Chinese: There is less information about Chinese individuals' risk for AD in the context of the *APOE*4 allele than there is for African Americans. However, a study of 538 residents of Shanghai gives information that generally accords—with an exception—with conclusions of other studies of *APOE*4 and AD risk.[22] In this study, having a single E4 allele increased AD risk by a factor of 3.1. Two E4 copies increased AD risk by a factor of 57. The latter number is very high and almost certainly an artifact of the small sample size (only seven people had the E4/E4 genotype,).

Japanese: Several studies have evaluated AD risk and *APOE* status in Japanese populations. The best study, based on its large size and prospective design, followed 2,603 Japanese-American men for incidence of dementia.[23] There were flaws in the study, the most obvious being the absence of any female participants, and another being the limited number of participants with the E4/4 genotype. In this study, the odds of dementia for "any E4 genotype" (E3/E4, E2/E4, or E4/E4) was increased by a factor of 2.39 compared with E3/3 carriers. A smaller study (which included Japanese women) found the odds of dementia for men and women with one E4 gene to be increased by a factor of 2.4-5.6. Two E4 genes increased risk by a factor of 33.1.[24] (The

---

[22] Katzman R, et al. Effects of of apolipoprotein E on dementia and aging in the Shanghai Survey of Dementia. *Neurology*. 1997;49:779-785

[23] Havlik RJ, et al. APOE-E4 predicts incident AD in Japanese-American men: The Honolulu–Asia Aging Study. *Neurology*. 2000;54:1526–1529

[24] Farrer LA, et al. Effects of age, sex, and ethnicity on the Association Between Apolipoprotein E Genotype and Alzheimer Disease: a Meta-analysis. *JAMA*. 1997:278:1349-1356

latter number is unreliable and due to the small number of people with two E4 genes.)

Hispanics: Unsurprisingly, given the prevalence of the E4 effect on Alzheimer's disease risk in other ethnicities, the E4 gene also increases AD risk in Hispanics. Risk in Hispanics with one copy of the E4 gene is increased by a factor of 1.7-4.5, while two E4 genes increases risk by a factor of 2.3-12. The wide risk range for Hispanic E4/4 carriers suggests problems with the data set: as with Japanese and Chinese E4/4 carriers, there were only small numbers of Hispanic E4/4 carriers, and conclusions based on these small numbers are not as reliable as assessments of the much more numerous E3/4 genotype.[25]

In the context of a first-degree family history of AD, does the presence of the APOE4 gene increase risk still further? This is the final genetic situation we will consider. If a 1st-degree family history of AD increases AD risk, and if the APOE4 gene separately

[25] Rippon GA, et al. Familial Alzheimer Disease in Latinos: Interaction Between APOE, Stroke and Estrogen Replacement. *Neurology.* 2006 January 10; 66(1): 35–40. doi:10.1212/01.wnl.0000191300.38571.3e,

Farrer LA, et al. Effects of age, sex, and ethnicity on the Association Between Apolipoprotein E Genotype and Alzheimer Disease: a Meta-analysis. *JAMA.* 1997:278:1349-1356,

Tang M-X, et al. Relative Risk of Alzheimer Disease and Age-at-Onset Distributions, Based on APOE Genotypes among Elderly African Americans, Caucasians, and Hispanics in New York City. *Am. J. Hum. Genet.* 1996;58:574-584,

Maestre G, et al. Apolipoprotein E and Alzheimer's Disease: Ethnic Variation in Genotypic Risks. *Ann Neurol* 1995;37:254-259,

Tang M-X, et al. The APOE-e4 Allele and the Risk for Alzheimer's Disease Among African Americans, Whites, and Hispanics. *JAMA.* 1998;279:751-755

increases risk, then it makes sense that a normal person with both risk factors would have a dementia risk that is greater than the risk posed by either factor alone. Two studies conclude that people with the APOE4 gene and a family history of AD are 3-4.6 times more likely to develop AD than people without the APOE4 gene and with a family history of AD.[26][27]

Now consider a slightly different situation: a woman (who does not know her own *APOE* genotype) has a father with Alzheimer's disease *and* the *APOE*4 gene. What is the daughter's risk for AD? This may seem like an unlikely circumstance that isn't worth exploring. Soon, however, *APOE* genotyping will occur more commonly as genetic testing becomes increasingly available, particularly in the context of a workup of a demented family member. Children of demented parents will be presented with precisely this information: a parent with dementia and one or two copies of the E4 gene. What does this mean for the child?

The literature's the bottom line is that the combination of AD *and* the *APOE*4 gene in a first-degree relative with dementia increases the risk of AD for family members, and this risk is above and beyond the risk that is already posed by the family history of dementia. In one study, the increased risk to the first-degree

---

[26] Huang W, et al. APOE Genotype, Family History of Dementia, and Alzheimer Disease Risk. A 6-Year Follow-up Study. *Arch Neurol*. 2004;61:1930-1934

[27] Slooter AJC, et al. Risk Estimates of Dementia by Apolipoprotein E Genotypes From a Population-Based Incidence Study: The Rotterdam Study. *Arch Neurol*. 1998;55:964-968

relative was 18%.[28] Another study confirmed this finding and demonstrated the *APOE*4 dose effect: relatives of demented patients have a higher risk for dementia if their demented relatives have two E4 copies instead of just one.[29]

This chapter has covered a lot of complicated information. At this point you are probably experiencing data fatigue. Maybe you feel overwhelmed not only by the facts and numbers, but by the realities of dementia genetics, the in-your-face quality of the statistics, the talk of risks and probabilities that can seem self-fulfilling. Carol, too, grapples with the complexity of Alzheimer's disease genetics and the truths that they unearth. But she wants to understand them because she has a first degree relative with AD—her mother. Her experience in working through the genetic data may also help clarify the reader's own understanding of risk.

Carol and Millie: Family matters

Carol has at last become a patient. She gave in—she needed to ask for help in understanding whether her memory symptoms are normal for age or not. She isn't sure if her memory mistakes have increased, but it's possible. She's not old—she's only in

---

[28] Farrer LA, et al. Apolipoprotein E Genotype in Patients with Alzheimer's Disease: Implications for the Risk of Dementia Among Relatives. *Ann Neurol.* 1995;38:797-808.

[29] Martinez M, et al. Apolipoprotein E e4 Allele and Familial Aggregation of Alzheimer Disease. *Arch Neurol.* 1998;55:810-816

her mid-50s—but she's getting older, and it isn't impossible that she has early-onset Alzheimer's disease. She doesn't really believe that she has AD, but she has a mother with the disease, and this fact has changed how Carol feels about her own risk for dementia. Anyhow, she says to herself, if I don't have AD now, I'd like to know if I'm going to get it. She makes an appointment with a neurologist.

Cognitive testing reveals that Carol has a well-crystallized intelligence and negligible memory errors that are well within the range of normal. She does not have AD. Once told the good news, it's clear that she expected it, "But it's good to hear it from the doctor." Her blood testing is normal. She even gets a brain MRI, which she and the neurologist look at together. Her brain looks completely normal. It's plump, says the neurologist. That's good.

They move on to discuss her risk for AD given her mother's diagnosis. Seeing her need for information, the neurologist, who is writing a book for patients about dementia, suggests that she read the chapter entitled, "What a Family History of Dementia Means for You." They can then discuss questions she might have about the information or about her own cognitive prospects. Carol does her best with the material, but she has no scientific training and would like clarification on a few points. She emails the neurologist. (The following email exchanged has been edited for clarity.)

Carol: What does "lifetime risk" of dementia mean?

Neurologist: It is the risk of getting dementia over the entire span of someone's life. A "lifetime" is usually considered to be about 80-85 years. The longer the life, the greater the risk for dementia. If we knew that someone was going to die at age 50, then the risk for getting dementia over that short lifetime is pretty close to zero. But if someone lives to be 80, their risk for dementia is much higher.

C: You say that the "background risk" for getting dementia is 10-12%. What is "background risk"?

N: The background risk is the average risk for getting dementia among people who live into their 80s in the USA. A background risk of 10-12% means that if we took a group of 100 random people, 10-12 of them would get dementia by the time they are age 85.

C: But you say that some people's risk for AD is much higher. How can this be if the background risk is 10-12%?

N: 10-12% of all of people in the USA will get dementia. That's looking at *everyone*, but not everyone is the same. Within the USA are many smaller groups (sub-groups, we could say): adults, children, employed, unemployed, drivers, bicyclists, cinephiles, bibliophiles, tall people, bald people, people who speak two languages…We could think of thousands of possible groups. We could take one of these groups of people and follow them for 85 years and see how many of them get dementia. This would be pointless for most groups, because most groups (cinephiles) will not have a higher (or lower) chance of getting dementia than the background risk because there is nothing about watching movies, for example, that would affect a person's tendency to get dementia. Some groups, however—bicyclists, perhaps—could have a lower dementia rate than the background rate, because exercise reduces dementia risk. (I don't know if this is actually true for bicyclists. I am making this example up.) Alternatively, some groups may have a higher dementia risk. Having studied many groups of people, researchers have identified some of these higher-risk groups. Dementia risk varies according to gender, ethnicity, family history, and other genetic factors (for instance, the kind of *APOE* gene a person has). It is also increased by other factors: having high blood pressure, diabetes, heart issues, and strokes. So the more we know about an individual, the more precisely we can determine the risk for dementia.

C: So I have three things against me?

N: It's true that being a woman and having a parent with AD each increase your risk for dementia. What is the third factor you are thinking of?

C: I am African American. But I have to clarify this. My mother is African American, but my father was not. His family was from Italy but he said he also had some Russian in him. If my mother is African American and my father is White, what is my risk?

N: That's a good question. There is no good information about this specific situation. When researchers recruit "African Americans" for a dementia study, they simply ask people if they identify as African American. You identify as African American, and your father is White—so your background emphasizes the point that there is a lot of genetic diversity within a group of people who identify as a certain ethnicity. Another way to say this is that ethnic identity may not tell us very much about a person's genetics.

C: Ok. Then I'm not sure how to use my ethnicity in knowing my risk for AD. Maybe I just shouldn't consider it, because it doesn't look like there is any information here that applies directly to my background. Maybe I should just consider my gender and family history?

N: I think that is fine.

C: Then what would my risk be? I looked at [Table A at the end of this book] and think I understand it. If I look at the "Family History" column and then down to "Any Female", I see 43.9%. Is that correct?

N: That's correct.

C: That's bad! It's almost a 50% chance of getting dementia. This isn't the news I want to hear, Doctor! Tell me something good.

N: I understand! But there is a lot of room for optimism here. That's a big number, yes, but remember it includes all comers: *all* people who have a family history and are female. Remember earlier when we discussed "background risk"? That's the risk for everyone in the USA. But we know that not everyone in the USA has exactly the same dementia risk. Some people have more risk for dementia than others: a "background risk" of 10-12% is just the average of the dementia risk for everyone in the group. Some people's risk is higher than 10-12%, some people's risk is lower. The same thing applies to your group ("women" plus "people with a family history of dementia"). The number you see is just an average. Some people in your group have many other dementia risk factors: high blood pressure, high cholesterol, obesity, smoking, strokes, lack of regular exercise, alcoholism. Those people raise the overall risk for the group. Some people, like you, who have none of these problems, have a much lower risk for AD than the average. So although you can't do anything about gender or family history, there are dementia risk factors that you can control (blood pressure, etc). This is very good news.

The last thing I would say about this is something we haven't emailed about: the APOE gene. Among your group ("women" plus "family history of dementia") is the gamut of APOE genes: E2, E3, and E4. People with the E2 and E3 genes are less likely to get AD than those with the E4 gene. The E4 people in your group increase the average risk of AD for the entire group, just as people with high BP or diabetes do. But if you don't have the E4 gene then your risk would be lower than the group average.

C: I wanted to ask about the *APOE* gene. My mom didn't have the *APOE* test. Should she get it?

N: No. The test is most useful in estimating risk for dementia. Once a person has dementia, the test is no longer useful.

C: Do you think I should get the *APOE* test? Would you get the *APOE* test?

N: I had the test. My maternal grandmother had dementia (late onset). I can't tell about my mother yet. My father died quite young and so I do not know whether he would have had dementia. So I don't really have a first degree relative with dementia. But I asked for the test from my primary care doc because information helps me cope. I have always been concerned about the possibility of dementia, and I knew I would be better able to deal with worry whether the *APOE* test showed I had the E4 gene or not. For me, knowing is better than not knowing. I felt that if I had the E4 gene, it would just confirm what I had already guessed about my risk. And if I had the E3 gene then I would be happy to know that my risk is less than I imagined. It turns out that I have the most common genotype: two E3 genes. This means that my APOE gene neither increases nor decreases my risk for AD. That is reassuring to me.

Bottom line is that if learning you have the E4 gene would increase your dementia dread, then you shouldn't get the test. Having said that, the chance of having at one copy of the E4 is not high, about 25% or less (it depends on what study you read), and the chance of having two E4 copies is only about 3%. But the chance of having two E3 copies (which would mean that you have no increased risk at all from the *APOE* gene) is 54% or greater (again, depending on the study). The point is that most people have the E3 gene, and most people do not have an E4 gene.

If you are thinking about getting the *APOE* genetic test, then I would be happy to give you more information about the pluses and minuses of testing so you can make a good decision about whether to get it or not. Would you like this information?

C: I would. Will you send it to me?

🔔 REMEMBER:

✓ Worry that one might develop Alzheimer's disease (AD) is often based less on an accurate understanding of true risk and more on fears generated by vivid examples of dementia among family or friends.

✓ For most people, the true risk for AD is different than their perceived risk.

✓ Inherited genes can influence risk for AD. Beta amyloid (β-amyloid) is a substance that accumulates in the brain in abnormal quantities in AD, and genetic factors increase β-amyloid in the brain.

✓ A family history of AD more than doubles an individual's lifetime risk for AD.

✓ Other factors that influence an individual's lifetime risk for AD are gender, ethnicity, and *APOE* genotype.

✓ The *APOE* gene has three variants, or alleles: *APOE2*, *APOE3*, and *APOE4*. People with the *APOE4* gene tend to accumulate more β-amyloid in their brains, thus increasing their risk for Alzheimer's disease.

✓ Having one copy of the *APOE4* gene increases the lifetime risk for AD to 20-30%. Having two copies of the *APOE4* gene increases the risk to 50-60%.

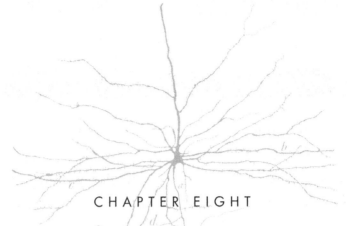

CHAPTER EIGHT

APOE GENETIC TESTING

▶ *APOE* genetic testing helps in understanding an individual's long-term prospects for cognitive health.

▶ Interpretation of *APOE* genetic test results requires an accurate understanding of *APOE* genetics and Alzheimer's disease.

▶ Obtaining *APOE* test results may improve emotional well-being, provide valuable information for family planning, and improve health behaviors.

▶ *APOE* testing may not be psychologically beneficial for people with anxiety or depression.

▶ *APOE* testing may or may not be right for you.

▶ *Read on to learn more.*

The information in the previous chapter about the *APOE* gene and its effect on Alzheimer's dementia risk would be useless if it weren't possible to test for the gene. Testing is indeed available; I've had the test myself. For the curious, the people for whom more information is better than less, who prefer facts to intuition, the test is appealing. Results give an individual a better sense of the possibilities for their cognitive future. Knowing one's *APOE* genotype, whether good (*APOE2* or *APOE3*) or bad (*APOE4*), neutralizes at least some of the factors that elicit dread, the "involuntary, delayed, unknown, uncontrollable, unfamiliar, potentially catastrophic, and severe."

Yet there is much handwringing among physicians about the propriety of *APOE* testing. While a few authors tentatively explore the advantages of testing, most oppose it. These same physicians do not hesitate to give patients other potentially difficult information about dementia risk. Recall our earlier discussion of Mild Cognitive Impairment, a diagnosis that is commonly given to the aged and forgetful. Most people with MCI do not progress to dementia: somewhere between 30-50% MCI cases revert to normal, and 37-76% remain cognitive stable and fail to progress to dementia. A diagnosis of MCI is therefore much worse at predicting dementia than *APOE* genetic testing, yet it is standard practice to diagnose MCI even in the absence of further counseling, available treatment, or regard for the psychologic consequences of the diagnosis. This is a double standard. On what basis is the utility of *APOE* genetic testing dismissed by physicians? Several objections to *APOE* testing are raised, and it is worth questioning their relevance to the individual keen to understand their risk for dementia.

The first objection to *APOE* testing is that interpretation of the results requires expertise. Proper counseling about the nature of the test and the meaning of results is necessary prior to testing. Such counseling minimizes the chance of an adverse psychologic reaction to results. But even with counseling, misunderstandings may persist in patients' minds due to the complexity of the information presented because "with complex conditions such as AD, where inheritance patterns are less precise, there is more latitude for personal interpretation of family history and disease risk."[1] These misunderstandings may have negative psychologic effects that outweigh any potential benefits of testing.

A second argument against *APOE* testing is the test's low sensitivity and specificity: a positive *APOE*4 test does not guarantee Alzheimer's disease, and negative test does not mean that a patient will not get AD. Why test if the results only create ambiguity?

A third argument submits that we have no intervention to offer *APOE*4 carriers to mitigate their dementia risk. Therefore, if testing does not change what the physician can do for the patient, testing is not appropriate.[2]

If the reasoning is overall sound, it is incomplete. Let's look at the third argument first: *If APOE testing does not change treatment*

---

[1] Hiraki S, et al. Perceptions of Familial Risk in those Seeking a Genetic Risk Assessment for Alzheimer's Disease. *J Genet Counseling.* 2009;18 (2), 130-136. DOI: 10.1007/s10897-008-9194-8

[2] Goldman JS, et al. Genetic counseling and testing for Alzheimer disease: Joint practice guidelines of the American College of Medical Genetics and the National Society of Genetic Counselors. *Genet Med.* 2011;13(6). DOI: 10.1097/GIM.0b013e31821d69b8

for the patient, then testing is not appropriate. In this context, treatment presumably means a medication, perhaps something like aducanumab, the drug approved by the FDA in 2021 for treatment of patients already diagnosed with AD. It is indeed true that no drug is available for prevention of AD in people who are without symptoms but who are at high risk for developing AD—for example, those with a 1ˢᵗ-degree family history of AD and/or who carry the *APOE4* gene. Yet physicians often test for disease (diabetes, high cholesterol) without the patient first committing to treatment. A positive test for high cholesterol, for instance, does not always entail a change in treatment for the patient because some patients decline treatment. Similarly, test results may be abnormal but not abnormal enough to require treatment. But physicians still do the test because it is better to know than not to know.

Another approach to the argument (*If testing does not change treatment for the patient, then testing is not appropriate*) broadens the notion of "treatment" to mean not just medication, but "benefit". After all, treatment with medication is only one means, among others, of producing a beneficial outcome for patients. Recall the discussion of "perceptions of personal risk": conditions that most frighten people are those that are perceived as "involuntary, delayed, unknown, uncontrollable, unfamiliar, potentially catastrophic, dreaded, and severe"—a concise description of the worries surrounding dementia. It follows that treatment of potential Alzheimer's disease includes mitigation of the psychologic aspects of contemplating the disease. Easing the anticipatory fear of AD is a therapeutic success and should be accepted as legitimate treatment.

Indeed, people who seek *APOE* testing understand that "treatment" for AD is limited, yet they pursue testing for other reasons that they consider equally valid. The neurologic literature can tell us a lot about why people seek *APOE* testing and about their response to test results. The REVEAL Study is a series of papers that examine the psychology of *APOE* testing in people with a family history of AD. The papers explore motivations for *APOE* testing, perceptions of pros and cons of testing, and reactions to *APOE* genotype results. According to the REVEAL study, the most common reasons for seeking *APOE* testing are to arrange personal affairs in case of AD, to prepare one's spouse or children for the possibility of AD, and in the hope that an effective AD treatment will be developed.[3] Positive *APOE*4 test results motivated one group of cognitively normal people to anticipate the practical difficulties posed by an AD diagnosis: comparing *APOE*4 negative to *APOE*4 positive people, the latter were 5.76 times more likely to purchase long-term care insurance.[4]

The REVEAL studies also show that many people benefit from *APOE* testing in strictly emotional ways, with some participants commenting that "knowledge is power" and acknowledging their need for information to feel control over situations: "for some the act of acquiring genetic information was seen as a way to confront their risk and therefore exert control. ... For some

---

[3] Roberts JS, et al. Reasons for Seeking Genetic Susceptibility Testing Among First-Degree Relatives of People With Alzheimer Disease. *Alzheimer Disease and Associated Disorders.* 2003;17(2):86–93

[4] Zick CD, et al. Genetic Testing For Alzheimer's Disease And Its Impact On Insurance Purchasing Behavior. *Health Affairs.* 2005;24(2):483-490. DOI: 10.1377/hlthaff.24.2.483

people knowing their genetic information may be a prerequisite for progressing on to other emotion-focused coping strategies."[5] The conclusion of this study is that "Even without prevention or treatment options, genetic testing may be a useful coping strategy for some at-risk individuals." *APOE* testing was beneficial for these individuals even in the absence of other treatment for AD.

Having good reasons for seeking testing, and having some positive responses to results, does not ensure that there aren't also some negative psychologic effects to learning one's *APOE* genotype. Is there a downside to testing? This question relates to the first two objections to *APOE* testing proposed above (*APOE test result interpretation requires expertise and proper counseling*, and *Having the APOE4 gene does not guarantee dementia, so why test?*). Both of these objections essentially state that, even with proper counseling, knowing one's *APOE* genotype has more potential for harm than good. Yet the REVEAL studies do not support this intuition. For example, a study of people with a parent with AD "measured symptoms of anxiety, depression, and test-related distress 6 weeks, 6 months, and 1 year after disclosure or nondisclosure" of their *APOE* genotype. Half of the participants were told their genotype and half were not, and there was no significant difference in anxiety, depression, or test-related distress among the two groups at any point in the study.[6] One year after learning their

[5] Gooding HC, et al. Genetic susceptibility testing for Alzheimer disease: Motivation to obtain information and control as precursors to coping with increased risk. *Patient Education and Counseling.* 2006;64:259–267

[6] Green RC, et al. Disclosure of *APOE* Genotype for Risk of Alzheimer's Disease. *N Engl J Med.* 2009;361:245-54

APOE genotype, these patients still felt that the pros of testing strongly outweighed the cons.[7]

This is not to say that all patients in the REVEAL study responded positively to testing; some patients found their *APOE*4 positive test results to be depressing, frightening, or disappointing, "but these feelings were not associated with clinically significant psychological distress." Moreover, "Baseline scores for anxiety and depression were strongly associated with post-disclosure scores of these measures"—that is, the participants who felt anxiety and depression after learning their *APOE* genotype were those who had anxiety and depression prior to testing, suggesting caution with testing in this demographic. Perhaps the worst possible outcome of *APOE* testing would be suicide. A few REVEAL participants gave their motivation for *APOE* testing as "to plan for suicide" in case of *APOE*4 positivity, but in follow-up interviews these people had changed their minds: they stated that while they would still consider suicide, they would do so only if symptomatic for AD, and they denied any suicidal thoughts provoked by the test result itself. It seems likely that these people changed their ideas about suicide because of the facts they learned about the *APOE*4 gene: they understood that having the E4 gene does not ensure AD but only increases risk.

Recall that about 25% of all people have one copy of the *APOE*4 gene and that only about 3% of all people have two copies of the gene. This means that most people who learn their

---

[7] Christensen KD, et al. Changes to perceptions of the pros and cons of genetic susceptibility testing after *APOE* genotyping for Alzheimer disease risk. *Genet Med* 2011:13(5):409–414.

APOE genotype are negative for *APOE*4 and do not have an increased *APOE*-associated risk for AD. For these people, the benefit of testing is more obvious: *APOE*4-negative patients are usually reassured by test results. On receiving an *APOE*4-negative result, one REVEAL study participant with a family history of AD reported that, "I feel less fearful. Although I understand my risk is not zero, is in fact two to three times greater than the risk of the average person, I have more confidence. Every time I, say, forget my keys, I don't think, 'Ah, this is how Alzheimer begins.'" Another *APOE*4-negative participant reported a new, quantifiable, and hence more realistic risk expectation after learning results: "Because my mother and her brothers have AD, I believed I had the *APOE*4 gene with a better than 50% chance of the disease. Now I believe my risk is at 25%, and I feel much more positive about the chances of not having AD. I no longer worry every time I have a memory glitch and am much calmer."

Even some of those who tested positive for the *APOE*4 gene in the REVEAL study found a benefit to testing. About half of all the participants felt relieved after receiving their *APOE* genotype, including some of the *APOE*4 positive participants, suggesting two possible explanations. First, participants' pre-test intuitions magnified their sense of risk, and their true risk, established by their *APOE* test results, seemed relatively low in comparison. Second, some participants described the therapeutic effect of knowing their *APOE* genotype. One participant stated, "The old adage is information is power…Being reasonable makes you feel strong. Actually you could call it doing sort of intellectual triage," while another stated that, "When it comes to genetic testing, I mean, one doesn't really have any control at all. Except that information is control." For these participants, knowing was better than not knowing, even if their test results were unfavorable. The benefit of knowing, of seeing and understanding one's risk for AD, for the better or the worse, is the point suggested by Hannah Fry in the quotation at the beginning of this chapter: mitigating ambiguity has a therapeutic effect, and numbers, even if imperfect, are better than having no numbers at all.

Ultimately, parsing the arguments by physicians for or against *APOE* genetic testing is probably moot: the days are short for the physician or counselor as the genetic testing gatekeeper. It is now a simple matter for an individual to order testing through an online lab. It is reasonable to consider *APOE* testing if you understand the material in this chapter and have a good qualitative grasp of *APOE*'s effect on AD risk—the *APOE*4 gene is neither necessary nor sufficient to cause AD—plus a firm quantitative grasp of the implications of possible results: a single E4 copy increases risk by a factor of about 3-4 and two copies increases risk by a factor of about 8; the E3 gene has no effect on AD risk; and the E2 gene reduces dementia risk.

Testing may be right for you if results could inspire better control of blood pressure, diabetes, or cholesterol, or if testing prompts you to make long-term plans, from anticipating financial needs to preparing family for the possibility of your disability. After all, we make small, anticipatory financial commitments against risk—fire, flood, unemployment, or disability—that are much smaller than the risk conferred by the *APOE*4 gene, and having a clear-eyed, quantitative understanding of one's AD risk is an advantage in making wise decisions about one's family's future.

Before testing, imagine your response to a positive *APOE*4 genetic test, recalling that anxiety or depression can be exacerbated by testing. If you think that you will probably feel worse about your future knowing you are *APOE*4 positive, that you will more closely monitor your cognitive mistakes, and that your anxiety and sense of doom will increase, then you may decide against testing. If, on the other hand, "information is control" for you, and any test result will puncture your worry and decompress it, then testing may be worthwhile.

The thoughts of the REVEAL study participants, their reactions to their family history of AD, and their feelings about knowing their own *APOE* genotype are typical of many people's anticipation of Alzheimer's dementia. Some of the REVEAL testimonials are touching, revealing hidden, long-held beliefs of inevitable cognitive doom. Many participants have clearly sustained a kind of exhausting emotional isometric, sensing their fate but resisting it, anticipating memory loss, analyzing each cognitive misfiring for evidence of dementia; and the tension within them is intensified by their sketchy, intuitive, and imprecise understanding of AD genetics and their lack of good information about actual risk. It is remarkable, and hopeful, that such longstanding and habitual worry responds to mere information: educating the REVEAL participants on their true risk for AD—using the same facts as those presented in this book—unclenched their anxiety, with most of them feeling, even after a year, that the information had an overall positive effect on their outlook. I hope the information in this book does the same for the reader. In contrast to our intuitions, which see in Alzheimer's disease the "involuntary, delayed, unknown, uncontrollable, unfamiliar, potentially catastrophic, dreaded, and severe"—and hence the inevitable—we can understand that doom is not inescapable. The great majority of us, in fact, will not get dementia.

🔔 REMEMBER:

- ✓ Everyone has two copies of the APOE gene.

- ✓ The APOE gene comes in three varieties ("alleles").

- ✓ About 25% of all people have one copy of the APOE4 allele and 3% have two copies. A single E4 copy increases dementia risk by a factor of about 3-4 and two copies increases risk by a factor of about 8.

- ✓ About 90% of people have at least one copy of the E3 allele and 54% have two copies. The E3 gene has no effect on dementia risk.

- ✓ About 16% of people have at least one copy of the E2 allele, which reduces dementia risk.

CHAPTER NINE

COGNITIVE PRESERVATION

► Some dementia risk factors are modifiable for adults, some are modifiable for children, and some dementia risk factors cannot be changed.

► The single modifiable risk factor with the most potential to reduce dementia risk is physical inactivity.

► More speculative potential interventions include being socially active, treating depression and anxiety, challenging the brain with puzzles or games, or other strategies.

► *Read on to learn more.*

I s dementia preventable? Each year, hundreds of scientific papers are published that investigate some aspect of this question, including, but not limited to, the potential effect on dementia risk of sleep patterns, mood, diet, exercise, meditation, leisure activities, education, career, sexual orientation, musical aptitude, micronutrient intake, environmental exposures of all sorts, sociability, stress, latitude, income, alcohol use, hearing acuity, arthritis, back pain, body weight, or nasal bacteria. And this is a very short sampling of factors that researchers have scrutinized for their association with dementia. Furthermore, some factors are starting points for research into yet more specific dementia risk factors. For example, the literature on the implications of "diet" on dementia risk is a garden of forking paths, many of which eventually lead to an entire landscape of research on vitamins and "nutraceuticals."

Much of this dementia literature is poor in quality, speculative, ill-considered, and without useful application, or it exploits fear for the sake of notoriety. The latter strategy is used by a group that is financially invested in dementia: those who understand that people will spend lots of money to prevent dementia. The list of dementia opportunists includes the pharmaceutical and vitamin supplement industries, hobbyist health gurus, addled influencers who mistake their internet popularity for actual expertise, naturopathic practitioners profiting from nostrums, and shills for myriad quasi-medical products, from yoga mats to aromatherapy to colonics. These groups aim to profit from people's worry, and their potential profit is indeed immense: in 2017, approximately 64-242 million people worldwide had mild cognitive impairment.[1] A ornamental dab of science plus worry equals sales.

Unfortunately, dementia researchers' efforts unintentionally abet the dementia opportunists. Science's immense dementia database provides the dementia prevention industry abundant material with which to backfill claims of product efficacy. Just about any proposition can be supported by the scientific literature if poor data is used unscrupulously or if data is taken out of

---

[1] Jongsiriyanyong S, et al. Mild cognitive impairment in clinical practice. *American Journal of Alzheimer's Disease and other Dementias* 2018;33(8):500-507

context. And this is usually how the scientific database is used by those who seek to profit from people's worry for dementia.

So how is the average person to know which dementia prevention recommendations to accept? What products are truly effective in preventing dementia? There is simply too much information available, much of it poor in quality. How is one to separate the good advice from the bad? How does one reconcile disagreements between claims, interpret the statistics offered in justification of conclusions or product efficacy, or keep up with the ever-growing literature?

This chapter attempts to cut the Gordian knot. It gives simple, data-based answers and bottom-line information by examining just one paper from the dementia literature, "Dementia prevention, intervention, and care: 2020 report of the *Lancet* Commission."[2] This paper was chosen because: 1) it is recently published, 2) it is a meta-analysis (it summarizes and evaluates the methods, data, and conclusions of many other selected papers), 3) it is published in a journal with a reputation for good research and editorial oversight, and 4) the researchers' methods are clearly described.

The limited advice offered in this chapter will be enough for some. Others will want more detail, and for these readers the chapter includes a brief catalog of the more speculative dementia prevention strategies investigated by the dementia literature. This book is not about dementia prevention; it is intended for those who wish to understand whether their memory symptoms may be due to dementia. A thorough review of all aspects of dementia

---

[2] Livingston G, et al. Dementia prevention, intervention, and care: 2020 report of the *Lancet* Commission. *Lancet* 2020; 396: 413–46. DOI: 10.1016/S0140-6736(20)30367-6

prevention would require a separate book. Such books exist, though in this author's opinion it isn't necessary to read an entire book about dementia prevention—that is, if one is seeking recommendations based on good data. The very scope of such a book obliges authors to choose the comprehensive over the credible, inducing wide-ranging recommendations on dementia prevention that overextend the data, much of which is already shaky. Perhaps a better approach for readers who want to learn more about dementia prevention is to start their own literature review (consider it as exercise for the brain), beginning with the publications referenced in *The Lancet*'s bibliography.

The article "Dementia prevention, intervention, and care: 2020 report of the *Lancet* Commission. *Lancet* 2020" makes the case for twelve potentially modifiable dementia risk factors. This is not to say that these are the only dementia risk factors—we know family history and *APOE* genotype, for instance, also increase dementia risk—but that the featured risk factors are modifiable and are strongly associated with dementia. One cannot change genetic risk, but one can, for instance, control blood pressure. These are the twelve potentially modifiable risk factors:

Hypertension	Smoking	Less education
Hearning Impairment	Obesity	Depression
Physical inactivity	Diabetes	Low social contact
Excessive alcohol consumption	Traumatic brain injury	Air pollution

The inclusion of some items on this list makes sense given what we know about, for example, vascular dementia, which is caused by hypertension (high blood pressure), diabetes, and smoking. Other items, such as hearing impairment, may provoke skepticism. Some items are truly modifiable, while others (air pollution) are clearly beyond an individual's ability to change.

Here are the same factors re-organized by modifiability.

Modifiable for the Adult	Modifiable for the Children	Not Modifiable
Hypertension	Education	Air pollution
Diabetes	Traumatic brain injury	
Obesity	Hearing impairment	
Physical inactivity		
Smoking		
Depression		
Low social contact		
Excessive alcohol consumption		

The list on the left is the to-do list for the adult who wishes to minimize dementia risk. We will discuss the middle column in a moment, and let's set aside "air pollution" altogether as a factor over which the individual has much control. The "Modifiable for the Adult" list may seem long, but we can simplify it by noting that four, and maybe five, of the elements may be treated by a single health behavior change: aerobic exercise. Exercise will improve and possibly resolve high blood pressure, diabetes, and obesity, and there is a good chance that it will improve depression. That leaves only smoking, low social contact, and excessive alcohol consumption on the to-do list.

The benefits of quitting smoking should be abundantly obvious to everyone by now, and this chapter will not belabor it. Whether low social contact is a cause of dementia, a manifestation of it, or just a non-causal marker for other risk factors (depression, hearing impairment, physical inactivity, excessive alcohol consumption, or some other factor) is a reasonable question. Alcohol use and its link to dementia is a complicated subject, with good evidence indicating that a certain amount of alcohol use protects against cardiovascular disease and dementia, and other evidence demonstrating that "excessive" use increases risk for these conditions. The *Lancet* article reports that 21 units of alcohol per week is excessive. This is helpful, to an extent—but the paper also notes that a "unit" of alcohol is not standardized and that the literature uses "a variety of definitions" for a unit. Keeping it simple, we can call one alcoholic drink "one unit," understanding that a heavy pour of wine or whisky is not one unit merely because it fits in a single glass.

Based on the *Lancet* paper, if there is one behavior that most people could change that would significantly impact their dementia risk it would be to increase their weekly amount of aerobic exercise. But no one wants to be told to exercise more, even when the stakes are as high as losing one's mind. So how much exercise is the least amount that will still prevent dementia? The answer is: more. Most people do not exercise at all. Most people, therefore, would benefit by almost any amount of exercise, such as one of the following activities three times per week (for 20 minutes, without stopping): brisk walking, jogging just faster than walking pace, bicycling on level ground, or swimming. When you are finished exercising, you should be out of breath and tired but not gasping. This is how you know you have properly exercised: if you are tired and out of breath after the activity. If you are not tired and out of breath, then you have merely moved your body around without effectively exercising it. If you are already an exerciser, then do a little more: increase your time to 30 minutes or your frequency to four or five times per week. If you follow through with regular exercise, making it a habit, your brain will live longer and your children may not have to care for a demented parent.

Is there something else that a parent with a concern for dementia can do for their children? This question brings us to the middle column of dementia risk factors, "Modifiable for Children." *The Lancet* identifies two, and maybe three, childhood risk factors that parents are in the position to influence: education, avoiding brain injury, and preventing hearing loss. At minimum, "education" means completing high school, but in terms of dementia prevention, more education—like more exercise—is better. There is a notion of "cognitive reserve," whereby education and other regular mental exercise enlarge the cognitive reservoir, which is drawn upon in later life to compensate for the cognitive diminishments of age. The greater the cognitive reserve the less likely one will develop abnormal cognitive symptoms. Education is the best way of increasing cognitive reserve, and many studies show that more educated people are less likely to develop dementia. A high school education is good, but a college education grants still more protection against dementia. It is also, perhaps, a comfort that a family's financial sacrifice for college buys not only a proper education but also a kind of cognitive equity. Long after you are gone and your child enters late middle age, your investment in college will continue to protect your child against dementia.

Mitigation of the final two early life dementia risk factors requires only commonsense safety measures. Ensure your child wears a helmet when bicycling, skateboarding, skiing, snowboarding, or doing any other activity that risks head injury, because brain injury is strongly associated with increased dementia risk later in life. Finally, hearing loss is associated with dementia. *The Lancet* suggest that improving hearing with hearing aids may protect against dementia, but it seems more likely that the statistical association between hearing loss and dementia is not causal. Nevertheless, ear protection is a good idea, whether young or old, and there is no harm in including it in this list of preventive health measures.

There is more to say about each of these, and other, dementia risk factors and prevention strategies, and readers may protest, "But what about...?" A detailed discussion of all risk factors and potential preventive measures is beyond the scope of this book. Researchers, examining myriad factors for their potential correlation with dementia, are like energetic seekers of needles in haystacks—with the drawback that often the hay is mistaken for needles either by researchers or readers. Research findings can be appealing, sensational, or news-worthy in their particularity (aromatherapy prevents dementia), counterintuitiveness (wearing hearing aids averts dementia), sunny optimism (goji berries strengthen the brain—and prevent cancer!), or in their confirmation of what has become accepted lore (doing crossword puzzles protects against dementia). In truth, selecting a risk factor or prevention strategy from this array of options is less a medical intervention then a lifestyle choice, fostering a feeling of healthiness that is reassuring and gives a sense of control over the fate of one's brain. This feeling of healthiness may not correlate with actual efficacy in preventing dementia, but for some people the mere possibility of a prevention effect and the reassurance of doing at least something, are enough to motivate adoption of a recommendation. For these readers the following list of possibly effective dementia prevention measures—each with variable degrees of support from the dementia literature—is included.

> Read
> Challenge your mind with learning something new
> Be social
> Get the flu vaccine
> Eat a Mediterranean diet
> Eat a DASH diet (Dietary Approaches
> to Stop Hypertension)
> Eat a MIND diet (Mediterranean-DASH
> Intervention for Neurodegenerative Delay)
> Ensure good sleep
> Treat depression
> Manage stress

Talk of dementia risk factors may prompt some readers to make two lists in their heads—one containing the dementia risk factors they have, and the other the factors they do not have—and feel reassured if the latter list is longer than the former. It is undeniably a good sign if one has only a few or no dementia risk factors, but caveats apply. The first caveat is the fact that disease risk factors do not affect all individuals in the same way. For example, some lifelong smokers never develop cancer, heart attacks, or dementia, while some nonsmokers may have these problems even when young. Additionally, the actual risks for dementia posed by such factors as hypertension and diabetes probably vary according to how well these problems are controlled. The dementia risk to a person whose blood pressure is well-controlled with medication is less than that of someone with persistently high blood pressures, although both people carry a diagnosis of hypertension. The third caveat regarding *The Lancet's* list is that each item poses a different degree of risk. For instance, if everyone stopped smoking then *The Lancet* reports that the prevalence of dementia would be reduced by 5%, while ending air pollution would reduce dementia prevalence by only 1%. Abolishing hypertension or alcohol use would reduce prevalence of dementia by 2% and 1% respectively. Not all risk factors pose equal risk.

And finally, if you are reading this book and are middle-aged or older, I offer a candid fact: your dice are already half cast. *The Lancet* found that better education for the young would reduce dementia prevalence by 7%. The study identified no other single risk factor with as much potential for dementia prevention. Yet for the reader of this book, the opportunity to reduce this risk is largely past, just as we cannot take back the food we have eaten, the wine we have drunk, the cigarettes we have smoked, and the time we have spent alone or depressed. Perhaps it is a relief that after middle age some risks cannot be reversed; there is only so much dementia intervention still available, and we should not over-stress ourselves in pursuing interventions fruitlessly. We can only do our best to load the dice, and then we watch them roll.

My advice: simplify, and give yourself a break. Dementia prevention isn't a complicated jigsaw puzzle with hundreds of pieces, all of which must be properly placed or the problem isn't solved. Only the ten biggest pieces are really needed. Ten pieces are more than enough to manage, and the rest of the puzzle is really just minor peripheral stuff. If you read about a newly discovered dementia risk factor, don't immediately reproach yourself if it seems to apply to you, because anxiety is unwholesome for the older brain. If there are dementia risk factors that you simply cannot change, put them aside in your mind. If a book, for example, prescribes a lengthy list of prevention strategies, don't pursue all of them if doing so causes stress.

Instead, be realistic and follow as many recommendations as you can, favoring those that pass the commonsense test (using hearing aids to prevent dementia fails this test), and ignoring those that are implausible (cultivating new nasal bacteria reduces dementia risk). Know that counterintuitive or extravagant new claims often have very short lifetimes before science firmly discredits them. Be aware of the dementia profiteers (pharmaceutical companies, nutraceutical companies, naturopaths, quasi-medical device salespeople) whose aim is to monetize worry by mis-representing science. And remember that much sensational news about dementia is unreliable if not outright dishonest.

And what if the odds are against us and we do get Alzheimer's disease? What then? How certain are we that a demented life is not worth living, and how can we know this? The last chapter in this book questions the premise that it is better to be cognitively normal than demented, exploring the question: Is it really so bad to be demented?

🔔 REMEMBER:

✓ Opinions and data on dementia prevention abound. Most are not based on reliable data.

✓ A 2021 publication by *The Lancet* is a trustworthy summary of some of the best dementia prevention studies and is the basis for this chapter's recommendations.

✓ Some dementia risk factors cannot be modified: age, family history of AD, ethnicity, gender, *APOE* genotype.

✓ Some dementia risk factors are modifiable: high blood pressure, diabetes, smoking, obesity, physical inactivity, excessive alcohol use, social isolation.

✓ The single modifiable risk factor with the most potential to reduce dementia risk in adults is physical inactivity. Increasing exercise reduces risk for dementia and mitigates other risk factors such as obesity, high blood pressure, and diabetes.

✓ In early life, increased education, avoiding brain injury, and using hearing protection are interventions that may reduce the lifetime risk of dementia.

✓ More speculative potential interventions include being socially active, treating depression and anxiety, challenging the brain with puzzles or games, and other strategies.

CHAPTER TEN

IS IT SO BAD TO
BE DEMENTED?

Millie still likes to be in the garden. Carol was never a gardener but now she gardens so her mother can still enjoy the tomatoes, snap peas, and flowers. She wears her mother's old apron, and in the pockets she found seed packets and a little notebook in which her mother once recorded yearly dates: the last frost, sowing starters in pots, planting starters in the garden, first fruit, first bloom, last cut flower, first frost. The handwriting is confident, clear and graceful. Carol is touched at this glimpse of her mother's previous mind. The year-to-year planning, the monitoring, the maintenance— the executive function, Carol remembers it's called. Her mother's mind was different then.

Carol is surprised at this thought. Instead of "My mother's mind was different then," shouldn't she have said, "My mother's mind is different now"? After all, Millie's pre-dementia mind was the original mind, that previous life the real and meaningful life, the benchmark, the one to which her new demented life ought to be compared. Isn't her mother's life now just a running out of the clock?

When Carol was more worried for her mind—before she saw the neurologist—she had ideas about how horrible dementia would be. But now, watching her mother in the garden, she has doubts. It may not be obvious to others, but Carol believes that Millie's life isn't without purpose. It isn't without pleasure. She isn't unaware of the world around her. She still takes an interest. It's a different quality of interest— she isn't taking notes any longer, she isn't collecting seeds for next season, she won't remember this year's first bloom—but it's real.

Millie sometimes sits on the couch and stares out the window. Anyone else would think that Millie's mind is vacant, but Carol knows that if she sits close enough she will hear her mother humming—usually As Time Goes By. *In these moments, Millie's expression is mysterious, and Carol can't tell what she is thinking, but she is sure that her mother—the person whose strong handwriting she reads in the notebook—is still somewhere inside. But perhaps Carol is reading too much into her mother's mind. Millie speaks less and less, and when she does her sentences are short and vague and lose their way. How can Carol really know what her mother is feeling?*

To those without dementia, a good life with dementia may be difficult to imagine. We have witnessed the demented's helplessness and frailty; the daily need for help with dressing and bathing and even for remembering their own selves; the sense that death is better than any such existence. We assume that cognitive impairment is incompatible with a good life.

But we assume too much. We underestimate the demented's capacity for adaptation, the cognitive abilities that they retain, and the pleasures that persist in their lives. In fact, if we bother to ask them, the demented will tell us that a demented life can still be worth living.

- ► Quality of life (QoL) decreases in old age whether one is demented or not.
- ► People with dementia rate their QoL higher than is expected by people without dementia.
- ► Cognition is unrelated to QoL in the demented.
- ► Both the demented and non-demented sustain QoL by adapting to adversity.
- ► *Read on to learn more.*

"For most of us, it would take a lot more than we think to make us permanently miserable."[1]

When I began research for this chapter, I didn't know the answer to the chapter title's question. But I had my hopes. While the realist in me questioned my own questioning of the premise that dementia is necessarily bad, the incipient dementia patient in me was optimistic, hoping to discover a counterintuitive truth in which dementia is just a rabbit hole to a different kind of contentment. I hoped the dementia literature would surprise me in showing that, despite appearances, dementia is a kind of purposeful shaping of an aged mind, a shedding of cognitive baggage no longer needed in old age. What if, I wondered, the loss of brain mass and synapses in the elderly brain—changes we incorrectly perceive as simply destructive—is instead a meaningful process of consolidation, a deliberate reworking of the brain's structure for a different cognitive purpose...

The realist awakes. The notion of a good side to dementia is absurd. Family members of dementia sufferers understand how bad dementia can be. It is inconceivable that there could be a positive side to the disease.

But let us step back from this intuition and look again. The certainty that the non-demented have that dementia is bad is not the same thing as knowing that dementia is bad for the demented. In other words, the non-demented should not assume they can speak to the quality of life for the demented. We look at a young person's energy and passion and we appreciate it; having experienced it ourselves, we can confirm that it is good. Yet had we not been young

---

[1] Riis J, et al. Ignorance of Hedonic Adaptation to Hemodialysis: A Study Using Ecological Momentary Assessment. *Journal of Experimental Psychology: General* 2005;134(1):3–9. DOI: 10.1037/0096-3445.134.1.3

once, it is possible that we would interpret youth's energy and passion differently—perhaps as a lot of unnecessary work and an excessive energy expenditure, or as purposeless or silly or trivial compared with the stability, pace, and quieter pleasures of maturity. We look at a demented person and cannot understand them—how could they be happy? In judging the quality of life of a demented person we must acknowledge that we lack the experience of having been demented ourselves. We have no special insight into what it may be like to be demented; we are ignorant in this respect. We legitimately empathize with dementia caregivers and the difficulties that dementia poses for them, but the experience of the demented themselves are not directly known to us. Can even we know that it is bad to be demented?

Moreover, the idea that the demented have it especially hard assumes that, in the absence of dementia, geriatric life is always good—an assumption that is plainly questionable. For most, old age is a struggle, whether demented or not. The aged are increasingly preoccupied with the maintenance of their failing bodies. For many of them, their lifeboat is sinking no matter how quicky they bail. No organ or tissue is exempt; leaks spring from all sides, and medical specialists rush about, plugging holes until, inevitably, the water pours over the rails.

In examining quality of life in dementia, therefore, our benchmark cannot be the quality of life of young people but the quality of life of contemporaries of the demented—the aged. The question to consider is not, "Is it so bad to be demented?" but "Is it really worse to be demented than to be just old?"

This chapter will explore three ideas. The first is that quality of life declines after middle age regardless of whether one is demented or not. This is not to say that quality of life in later life is poor but just that it is not as high as in middle age, and it is against this background that we should examine the quality of life of the demented. The second idea is that although people have a strong sense of their own quality of life, they are not good at judging the quality of life in other people. People with disabilities (such as paraplegia, kidney failure, or dementia) usually estimate their quality of life as much better than do witnesses without these problems. And the third idea explored by this chapter is that, despite the intuitions of people without dementia, many people with dementia (not all, but probably the majority) rate their own quality of life as good.

A final theme that runs throughout this chapter is the resourcefulness of human adaptation to the physical changes of life. Body changes are a fact of life at all stages, from infancy on. The physical changes that occur at each stage of life entail their own difficulties and benefits. Humans are flexible in confronting these changes, finding the good in life, the enjoyable, and making these positive aspects central to the experience of their own lives even in adversity, even with serious setbacks to their health—and even when witnesses interpret their quality of life as poor and life as not worthwhile. People find the good in life even after setbacks that are, in anticipation, self-evidently devastating.

HOW DOES QUALITY OF LIFE CHANGE OVER A LIFETIME?

"Quality of Life" is similar to happiness, well-being, or life satisfaction. Good QoL is the sense of one's life as enjoyable and worthwhile, while poor QoL is the feeling that one's life is hollow, unrewarding, and on balance a hardship or displeasure.

Some researchers say that quality of life over the lifespan looks like the graph below. (In this case, the researchers used the term "wellbeing.")[2]

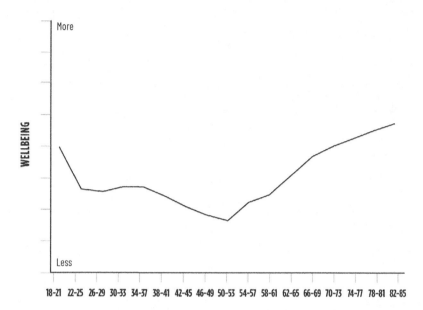

Figure 1: One version of well-being and age: the U-shaped curve

(Adapted from: Stone AA, et al. A snapshot of the age distribution of psychological well-being in the United States. PNAS 2010;107(22):9985–9990)

In this conceptualization, well-being is lowest at middle age due to the stress and worry of working plus the difficulties of child-rearing. Well-being's subsequent climb in late middle age is driven by retirement and the independence of children.

But this probably isn't what lifetime quality of life really looks like. The data used to make this curve is "cross-sectional"—the participants were asked to assess their QoL only once. Individual responses

---

[2]   Stone AA, et al. A snapshot of the age distribution of psychological well-being in the United States. *PNAS* 2010;107(22):9985–9990

were then plotted, and the dots connected. But this method gives only a snapshot of QoL at a single moment in time. What we really want to know is how an individual's QoL changes over a lifetime, so we should track individuals' QoL over their lives and then combine the results into a single curve—a "longitudinal study." Longitudinal studies of QoL in the non-demented show the opposite of Figure 1's U-shaped curve; they reveal an "inverted U-shaped curve," which peaks at about mid-life and is idealized here in Figure 2:[3]

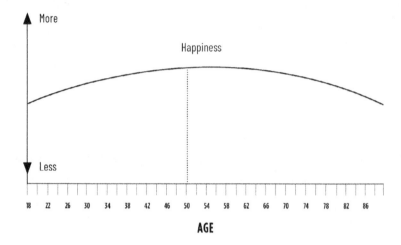

Figure 2: Another version of happiness and age: the inverted U-shaped curve

(Adapted from: Richard Easterlin. Life cycle happiness and its sources. Intersections of psychology, economics, and demography. Journal of Economic Psychology 2006;27:463-482.)

Why the increase in happiness to middle age and the decrease thereafter? If we take this curve apart and look at the more basic

---

3   Richard Easterlin. Life cycle happiness and its sources. Intersections of psychology, economics, and demography. *Journal of Economic Psychology* 2006;27:463–482. DOI: 10.1016/j.joep.2006.05.002

elements of happiness (satisfaction with family, job, finances, health), we see that happiness is an average of several unique lifetime trends.

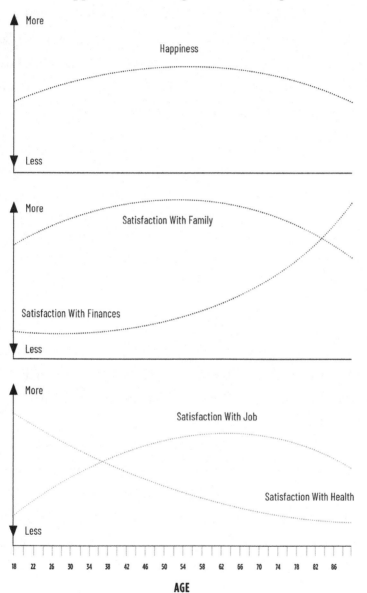

Figure 3: Life satisfaction elements and age

(Adapted from: Richard Easterlin. Life cycle happiness and its sources. Intersections of psychology, economics, and demography. Journal of Economic Psychology 2006;27:463–482.)

The first curve ("Happiness") is the average of all the curves below it. The combination of satisfaction with "Family," "Finances," "Health," and "Job" is an arc of happiness that rises from adolescence, peaks in middle age, and declines in the last half of life.[4] As an explanation for these curves, the author of this study describes how these life domains— satisfaction with family life, finances, job, and health—interact over the lifespan:

> Until people are around age 50 increased satisfaction with family life and work outweigh diminished satisfaction with health and contribute, on average, to a mild rise in happiness. From midlife onward, decreasing satisfaction with family life and work join that in health in causing a decline in happiness. This negative impact is considerably offset, however, by increasing satisfaction of people with their financial situation.

Of all the domains graphed above, we see that satisfaction with health is the most consistent, declining almost linearly from age 18 onwards. According to these graphs, health remains an important influencer of satisfaction late in life, when intractable health problems accumulate.

If health is an important influencer of quality of life, let us now look at how late-life illness affects QoL in the absence of dementia. Comparison with this group—the aged and the ill— will tell us whether dementia is especially disruptive of QoL or whether, instead, dementia is just one of many equally potent influencers of QoL in late life.

---

[4] Note that this study surveyed only people in the United States.

WHAT DOES QUALITY OF LIFE LOOK LIKE IN THE ELDERLY NON-DEMENTED?

Many aged people belong among the "multimorbid," those having at least two chronic diseases. Multimorbidity is reported in 55-98% of older persons, and the older someone is the more likely they will become multimorbid.[5] The list of conditions most commonly associated with multimorbidity includes arthritis, blindness, cancer, cardiovascular disease, diabetes, hearing problems, orthopedic problems, paralysis, amputation, spinal cord injury, head injury, obstructive pulmonary disease, chronic pain, and addiction/mental illness.[6][7] It would therefore be reasonable to expect that the multimorbid's quality of life suffers more than those with fewer medical conditions,[8] and that QoL drops in older age (because the number of health problems increase later in life). Indeed, if we take the second half of life (age 50 onwards), we see the decline in QoL that would be

[5] Marengoni A, et al. Aging with multimorbidity: A systematic review of the literature. *Ageing Research Reviews* 2010;10:430–439

[6] Cutler DM, et al. Measuring the Health of the U.S. Population. *Brookings Papers on Economic Activity. Microeconomics*, 1997, pp. 217-282. https://www.jstor.org/stable/2534757

[7] Albrecht GL, et al. The disability paradox: high quality of life against all odds. *Social Science & Medicine* 1999;48: 977-988

[8] Makovski TT, et al. Multimorbidity and quality of life: Systematic literature review and meta- analysis. *Ageing Research Reviews* 2019;53:100903. DOI: 10.1016/j.arr.2019.04.005

expected if we just looked at the second half of the curve of Figure 2, above:[9]

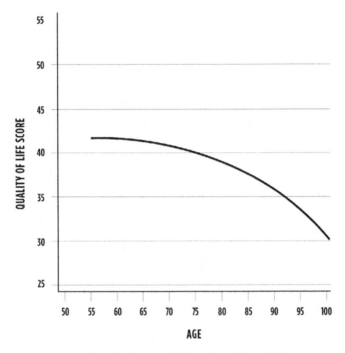

Figure 4: Quality of life declines after middle age

(Adapted from: Zaninotto P, et al. Age trajectories of quality of life among older adults: results from the English Longitudinal Study of Ageing. Qual Life Res 2009;18:1301–1309.)

This graph demonstrates a downward march in QoL from age 50 onwards. The rate of decline—the slope of the line—actually increases in later age as the number of medical problems and disability increase. The older someone is, the more medical problems they have. The more medical problems a person has, the worse their quality of life.

---

[9] Zaninotto P, et al. Age trajectories of quality of life among older adults: results from the English Longitudinal Study of Ageing. *Qual Life Res* 2009;18:1301–1309. DOI 10.1007/s11136-009-9543-6

ADAPTATION

Considering the challenges of old age, one might wonder why QoL does not decline even more. Why doesn't the QoL curve drop even more dramatically in late life? Consider Figure 2 again.

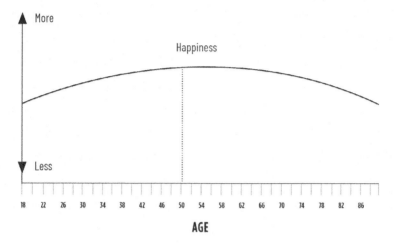

Figure 2: Another version of happiness and age: the inverted U-shaped curve

(Adapted from: Richard Easterlin. Life cycle happiness and its sources. Intersections of psychology, economics, and demography. Journal of Economic Psychology 2006;27:463-482.)

If we take the symmetry of this arc literally, we conclude that quality of life at 86 is about as good as it is at age 18. Old age has its advantages—financial stability, leisure, no work or child-rearing stress—but it makes no sense that QoL is the same at each end of the curve. If 86-year-olds were asked the question "Is your QoL the same now as when you were 18?" it is doubtful that any of them would answer "yes."[10]

---

[10] While many studies have investigated elderly QoL, I found no study that asked elderly subjects to compare directly their current QoL with early adulthood QoL. When asked about their QoL, elderly people generally compare their circumstances with those of people their own age, a tendency called "age norming".

So, although the QoL curve declines in old age, it is surprising that it does not decline more than it does. One study of the aged and multimorbid found that 93% reported moderate to severe disability. If health status directly determines QoL, then one would expect that 93% of the multimorbid participants in this study would report poor QoL. In fact, over half of them (54.3%) reported an excellent or good QoL.[11]

This paradox is also illustrated by a study of happiness among 22 Illinois State Lottery winners, 22 controls, and 29 people paralyzed in accidents.[12] Despite their unexpected good fortune, lottery winners were not happier than controls, suggesting that happiness has a "set point" from which it may be deflected by events but, eventually, returns to equilibrium. But there was another finding in the study that is especially relevant to this discussion. Permanently paralyzed people, despite their severe limitations, still rated their happiness above average: on a scale of 1-5, they rated "current happiness" as 2.96. Furthermore, paralyzed people rated "past and anticipated future happiness" higher than either controls or lottery winners, and they rated their enjoyment of "ordinary pleasures" (talking with a friend, watching television, eating breakfast, reading a magazine, buying clothes) higher than did lottery winners. Extreme fortune, for better or for worse, has a disproportionately low impact on actual QoL.

---

[11] Albrecht GL, et al. The disability paradox: high quality of life against all odds. *Social Science & Medicine* 1999;48: 977-988

[12] Brickman P, et al. Lottery Winners and Accident Victims: Is Happiness Relative? *Journal of Personality and Social Psychology* 1978;36(8): 917-927

Similarly, another study evaluated quality of life in people with kidney failure requiring hemodialysis (HD).[13] In chronic kidney failure, HD is required about three times per week. Treatment requires traveling to an HD clinic, where patients sit for several hours as the HD machine normalizes their blood electrolytes. Missing dialysis causes delirium; stop dialysis altogether and death is inevitable. To those with normal kidney function, life on HD appears poor. Yet comparing 49 healthy controls with 49 HD patients demonstrated no significant difference in mood. The study concluded that

> Hemodialysis patients do, largely at least, adapt to their condition. Although they report their health as being much worse than that of healthy controls, they do not appear to be much, if at all, less happy than people who do not have kidney disease or any other serious health condition.

The fact that mood did not suffer despite the limitations of life on hemodialysis indicates that our assumptions about what determines QoL are wrong. "It is possible," the authors comment, "that in coping with their hardship, patients have developed a tendency to focus more on positive experience. This may be a crucial part of the adaptation process."

This suggests that the elderly end of the QoL curve may be determined not merely by satisfaction with family, work, finances, and health. There are adaptive mechanisms that brace

[13] Riis J, et al. Ignorance of Hedonic Adaptation to Hemodialysis: A Study Using Ecological Momentary Assessment. *Journal of Experimental Psychology:* General 2005;134(1):3–9. DOI: 10.1037/0096-3445.134.1.3

the happiness curve and prevent it from declining to the extent that younger onlookers might expect. A deep dive into the psychology of adaptation to adversity is not necessary here, but the following quotations from the literature describe techniques used by people in adapting to health challenges.

- They may "accept their loss and adopt a positive attitude by trying to make the best of it and enjoy life."[14]

- "Their standards of evaluation may shift somewhat to accommodate [challenges] and to preserve feelings of well-being."

- They may "change the relative importance of life goals to emphasize goals over which more control can be exerted...[and place] importance on other life domains that are not impaired."[15]

- They employ "cognitive reappraisal," "a mechanism that refers to the reinterpretation of emotional information so as to alter its impact."[16]

- Individuals "view their lives as pleasant by retaining positive emotions and minimizing negative emotions."[20]

Our responses to medical adversity can be complex and counterintuitive and are a testament to the resourcefulness, optimism,

---

[14] Steeman E, et al. Living with dementia from the perspective of older people: Is it a positive story? *Aging & Mental Health*. 2007;11:2, 119-130. DOI: 10.1080/13607860600963364

[15] Ready RE, et al. Patient versus informant perspectives of Quality of Life in Mild Cognitive Impairment and Alzheimer's disease. *Int J Geriatr Psychiatry*. 2004; 19: 256–265

[16] El Haj M, et al. "La vie en rose": A positive shift of autobiographical memory in Alzheimer's Disease. *Archives of Gerontology and Geriatrics* 2020; 86:103953. DOI: 10.1016/j.archger.2019.103953

imagination, and stubbornness of the human mind. The worst events—anticipated, feared, disabling, and life-changing medical tsunamis—have their expected moment of impact and subsequent trauma, but eventually, it seems, the water recedes, and the disaster is discounted by the victim. Suffering is perceived as relative, disability is accommodated, and expectations are re-calibrated. People with dementia do this, too, as we will see in a moment.

If we are honest, these adaptive techniques probably feel familiar to most of us. We use at least some of them regularly in dealing with difficulties, even if we do so unconsciously. When travel plans are abandoned due to a pandemic, we are grateful for a "staycation." When a new job does not earn as much money as the old job, we increase our valuation of the new job's easier commute. Parents overwhelmed by a newborn baby feel better when they see the difficulties of parents with twins. In using these techniques of adaptation, we are not fooling ourselves into believing that we feel differently than we do. We are not papering over a true, deeper feeling with a false counter-narrative. Such an interpretation of adaptive techniques misperceives their actual work, which is to recalibrate fundamentally, to reframe, to reconcile expectations with circumstances in a way that is deep and psychologically authentic. Quality of life is fungible for humans. It is only to the onlooker that the process appears false and futile. And onlookers, we will learn, have notoriously poor judgement in estimating the quality of life of people with dementia.

CAN THE UNDEMENTED KNOW WHAT IT IS LIKE TO BE DEMENTED?

Though it is vast, the quality of life literature demonstrates, trial after trial, that when "proxies"—family or caregivers of the demented—are asked to assess the quality of life of the demented person in their care, they report lower QoL than do the demented themselves.

This disagreement between proxy and patient reporting of QoL has been called the "disability paradox," which is twofold: first, the disabled acknowledge serious limitations yet also report good to excellent quality of life (as we saw in the case of hemodialysis and paralyzed patients); "and, second, the general public, physicians and other health care workers perceive that persons with disabilities have an unsatisfying quality of life."[17]

One explanation for the disability paradox is simple: people project their own mental states on others. Caregivers' assessment of QoL in the demented are strongly influenced by their own psychologic status: caregivers' own depression and care burden consistently correlate with their assessment of low QoL in the patient. Even the type of shift that caregivers are working can influence their assessment of the QoL of the demented: night shift caregivers rate QoL in people with dementia lower than do day shift caregivers.[18] The QoL of caregivers may deteriorate as

[17] Albrecht GL, et al. The disability paradox: high quality of life against all odds. *Social Science & Medicine* 1999;48: 977-988

[18] Crespo M, et al. Factors associated with quality of life in dementia patients in long-term care. *International Psychogeriatrics.* 2013;25:4,577–585. DOI: 10.1017/S1041610212002219

a consequence of caring for their family member with dementia, but the demented's own QoL follows a different course.

Besides caregivers' projection of their own unhappiness on people with dementia (PWD), there is another explanation for the disability paradox. It represents a simple failure of imagination. Proxies simply cannot imagine that QoL could be preserved given PWD's disabilities, whose severity and progression they witness firsthand and daily. Proxies, of course, are comparing the PWD to themselves. Proxies are not answering the question, "How do you rate the QoL for the PWD?" but instead, "How would you rate your own QoL if you had a demented person's disabilities?" This error has been called a "scale of reference bias," whereby reference points that make sense for one group of people do not make sense for another, as explained in a study of adaption, scale of reference bias, and QoL:

> If you are asked about your well-being you do so by comparing yourself to people in a similar situation as yourself (friends, relative, people of your age, people with similar education, etc.), or by comparing the sources of your well-being with those of others people with more health problems than yourself (people without a job, people with a low income, etc.). The finding that patients with diabetes report relatively high levels of well-being may be because they compare themselves to other patients in a similar physical condition, or they may compare themselves to the situation they had expected themselves to be in at that stage of their disease.[19]

---

[19] Wim Groot. Adaptation and scale of reference bias in self-assessments of quality of life. *Journal of Health Economics* 2000;19:403–420. DOI: 10.1016/S0167-6296(99)00037-5

Proxies compare the quality of life of people with dementia to the QoL of younger, undemented, healthier people. This is misguided in many ways, not least because QoL diminishes with age regardless of whether one has cognitive problems or not.

In anticipating some potential catastrophe of health, finances, property loss, or family, (or dementia), our imaginations falter. We focus on what may be lost and overlook what remains, seeing mostly what will change as the result of a setback and ignoring what will not.[20] We observe the life of a person on hemodialysis and notice only the restriction and inconvenience, while the person on HD sees what is preserved. We observe that a demented person cannot drive, but we do not see the daily pleasures—sharing a meal, listening to music, going for a walk, watching TV, talking with a friend—that are still enjoyed.

In a way, this is encouraging: our intuitions, our fears, about what it is like to be demented have no power to anticipate the actual experience of dementia. Stated another way, we cannot rely on our fears, however powerful they may be, as accurate indicators of what it is actually like to live as a demented person. As we have seen, when the non-demented make judgements about the QoL of the demented, they are almost always wrong. Only the demented can tell us whether it is so bad to be demented. But we don't usually ask the demented whether their lives are as

---

[20] Riis J, et al. Ignorance of Hedonic Adaptation to Hemodialysis: A Study Using Ecological Momentary Assessment. *Journal of Experimental Psychology:* General 2005;134(1):3–9. DOI: 10.1037/0096-3445.134.1.3

difficult as we judge them to be. If we do bother to ask them, we get an unexpected answer: in dementia, QoL is often preserved.

Carol and Millie: Not so bad

Millie enjoys food. This certainly has not changed. She isn't picky, enjoying whatever Carol prepares. Carol cleans up, and Millie doesn't say "thank you." She also seems to have forgotten the word "please."

Millie doesn't do much, but she seems to enjoy it. She sits in front of the TV for hours. Sometimes she watches the TV, sometimes she hums.

Carol puts simple puzzles on the table. Millie doesn't fit the pieces together; this task is either beyond her or of no interest. But she likes arranging the pieces, pushing them around with her fingertip until the picture appears—though exploded: the pieces are unconnected but each is in approximately the right spot. She solves the puzzle her own way.

In the time between lunch and dinner Millie sometimes becomes agitated. She paces and seems to be looking for something. Carol first thinks that her mother has to use the bathroom, but that isn't it. Carol tries sitting her down and putting tea in front of her. Sometimes this works, sometimes it doesn't. Carol plays music, or she puts a bowl of snap peas on the table and shows her mother how to remove the stringy part from the pod. All this takes time and patience. Carol has

hired a caregiver to look after her mother when Carol is at
work or needs time to herself.

Millie hums As Time Goes By *so often that Carol looks up the*
words to the song, thinking that her mother would like to
sing them. Carol sings the song, and her mother hums along
but doesn't join in.

Moonlight and love songs
Never out of date
Hearts full of passion
Jealousy and hate
Woman needs man, and man must have his mate
That no one can deny
It's still the same old story
A fight for love and glory
A case of do or die

The words have nothing to do with Millie's life now. If her
mother understands the words—though Carol isn't sure that
she does—why does she like the song so much? To Carol, the
words are treacly and nostalgic, and that was never her
mother's style. She watches as her mother hums, the mysteri-
ous expression on her face, and she wonders if her mother is
looking back at her younger life not with nostalgia but with
its opposite. Is she, in fact, pleased that she no longer wants a
heart "full of passion/Jealousy and hate" and need not partici-
pate in "the same old story/A fight for love and glory/A case of

do or die." Is this knowledge—this long perspective on youth's turmoil—what is behind Millie's mysterious expression?

The struggles of young life are nothing to Millie. Such passions do not concern her. Instead, Millie enjoys her garden, the dahlias, the weight of a bowl of freshly picked tomatoes on her lap, the smell of the tomato leaves on her hands, the taste of raspberries, the warm sun. A heart full of passion, jealousy and hate—is this really better that the simpler pleasures of Millie's sedentary life?

Carol then questions something she had taken for granted, thinking: How do I know that normal cognition actually adds to the pleasures of such simple sensory experiences as a garden, food, or music? Is there a limit to how much memory adds to experience? She doesn't know the answer but thinks the question is worthwhile.

CAN THE DEMENTED HAVE GOOD
QUALITY OF LIFE?

It is an unfortunate fact of life that, even if our brains age normally, we must still expect quality of life to diminish. QoL slopes downward through the geriatric years, in which we spend increasing energy contending with disease and frailty until, at some point late in life, our QoL is significantly poorer than at mid-life.

We would therefore expect the same or perhaps even a more dramatic decline in quality of life for the demented, but the medical literature does not agree that QoL declines for all PWD.[21] QoL in dementia is mixed. Some people with dementia report a decline in QoL while others say their QoL is unchanged. Some PWD even report improvement in their QoL. One study showed no change in QoL over two years either for the worse or the better,[22] while others have shown no change in QoL for about 13-27% of PWD. The point here is not to say that a specific and predictable percentage of the demented have good, bad, or unchanging QoL. The point, instead, is that the demented have the same potential for good or poor QoL that the undemented

---

[21] Some of the studies discussed in this section use proxy ratings of QoL because they examined severely demented PWD. The authors of these studies felt that proxy ratings would be more reliable than self-reports of QoL in these patients. While proxy studies have been demonstrated elsewhere in the literature to correlate poorly with PWD's own reporting of their QoL, proxy ratings always underestimate actual QoL, suggesting that the effect of the studies discussed in this section is more robust (ie, QoL may be better than reported).

[22] Van der Zon A, et al. Two-Year Course of Quality of Life in Nursing Home Residents with Dementia. *Am J Geriatr Psychiatry* 2018; 26:754–764. DOI: 10.1016/j.jagp.2018.01.202

have. (This is assuming that PWD have their basic needs met: food, shelter, safety, and regular interaction with other people.) Some people, demented or not, will see their lives as overall pleasurable and worthwhile, and others will see their lives, on balance, as containing more difficulty than pleasure.[23]

It should not therefore be a surprise to learn that elements that make for good or poor QoL in dementia are the same as those we consider important determinants of QoL for anyone, demented or not. In the dementia literature, some factors emerge that are repeatedly associated with good or poor QoL. Good QoL for people with dementia is usually associated with social engagement, independence, living with a partner, having contact with family, good health, and good mood. Poor QoL is associated most strongly with depression, poor health, pain, anxiety, and lack of social contact with friends or family. With respect to the most basic elements of QoL, the demented are no different than the undemented: no one wants to be depressed, anxious, lonely, or sick; everyone wants autonomy, regular contact with family and friends, and a good mood. It is to be expected that a good portion of all people, demented or not, will have a mix of these good and

---

[23] Some may wonder whether, given their diminished cognitive faculties, it makes any sense to ask people with dementia about their quality of life. It is possible that people with dementia cannot accurately report how they feel. But for the most part, PWD do indeed report reliably. Studies of PWD in care facilities and with mild to moderately severe dementia show that about 77% can reliably answer questions about their QoL. Some studies have shown that accurate self-reporting is preserved even in severely demented individuals with very low scores on cognitive testing. This chapter's discussion of QoL in PWD, therefore, is confined to people with mild to moderately severe dementia. Once dementia is very severe, it is no longer possible to assess QoL directly.

bad factors in their lives, and the specific mix in an individual determines one's overall QoL. Does having dementia mean that one is more likely to have poor QoL? The short answer is "no."

The minds of people with dementia, though diminished, can still adapt. People with dementia alter their expectations, amend their scale of comparison, focus on what they can still do rather than what they cannot, interpret events more positively, and change their goals. They find new purpose, however modest it may be. Or they just forget about their problems and simply try to enjoy themselves. The human mind is good at finding equilibrium, even in dementia. An author describes some strategies used by PWD to maintain value in their life: [24]

> Some of these strategies include minimizing, rationalizing, normalizing, or somatising[25] problems; affirming one's competencies; denying problems; avoiding confrontation; using humour; training memory; using memory aids; avoiding reflection; and accepting…Within the context of a disturbed identity, these strategies allow one to restore identity.

Can people really adapt this well to dementia? If they are able to adapt to not driving, the loss of independence, and the need for help with basic tasks, it is perhaps a different and more difficult challenge to adapt to the loss of intellectual power. After all, the concern at the heart of many people's fear of dementia is

---

[24] Steeman E, et al. Living with dementia from the perspective of older people: Is it a positive story? *Aging & Mental Health.* 2007;11:2, 119-130. DOI: 10.1080/13607860600963364

[25] Somatization is manifesting a psychologic experience as a bodily symptom. For instance, a person with anxiety may perceive tingling in the arms that is not due to a neurologic problem but entirely due to their psychologic unrest.

that they will lose the pleasures of reading, learning, conversation, and curiosity. In other words, they believe that having normal cognition is necessary to having good QoL, and that QoL must therefore decline with cognitive loss. This is intuitively true, and it seems radical to suggest otherwise, though there are precedents that argue the opposite. (Part of the pleasure of intoxication is its holiday from normal cognition.) Yet, as we have already learned, despite cognitive loss, QoL is maintained in most people with dementia. It might therefore be helpful for those of us worried for dementia if we were able to understand the relationship (or lack of it) between cognitive loss, specifically, and quality of life.

Many good studies have inquired about cognition and its effect on quality of life in the aged. These studies evaluate people with dementia by comparing cognitive test scores with scores of well-being. One study followed people with Alzheimer's disease and people without AD over two years, comparing change in QoL between the groups.[26] At baseline, the AD group reported better QoL than the normal group. After two years, the normal group was no more or less likely to have stable QoL scores than the demented—decline in cognition did not correlate with decline in QoL. "QoL scores were similarly stable over time for most residents with and without AD diagnoses and were sensitive to changes in health/functional status." This means that general medical health, and not cognitive decline, was the main determinate of QoL in old age.

---

[26] Qin Z, et al. Longitudinal Comparison of Stability and Sensitivity in Quality of Life Scores Among Nursing Home Residents With and Without Diagnoses of Alzheimer's Disease and Related Dementias. *Innovation in Aging* 2021;5(3):1–11. DOI: 10.1093/geroni/igab024

Another study used a finer comb to tease out the relationship between cognitive status and its potential effects on quality of life by comparing QoL in cognitively normal individuals with two other groups: people with mild cognitive impairment (MCI) and people with AD.[27] There was no ambiguity in the results, which found "no significant differences found between self-reported QOL from AD, MCI, and controls. Overall, scores were nearly identical for the three groups." It did not matter for quality of life whether a person had dementia, Mild Cognitive Impairment, or normal cognition.

While these are just two studies demonstrating lack of correlation between cognitive status and QoL, they are controlled studies, which are rare.[28] The many uncontrolled studies generally agree that QoL in dementia is not determined by cognitive status but rather by emotional factors and general medical status. There are certainly papers that argue the opposite—that QoL tracks downward with cognition—but they are a distinct minority and not better in quality than the papers cited here. The overall thrust of the literature is reflected in the following quotations, which, in the interest of "the whole brevity thing,"[29] are offered as a distillation of the literature.

> Well-being was directly predicted by mental health (anxiety and depression) and social relationships rather than by…global dementia severity[30]

---

[27] Ready RE, et al. Patient versus informant perspectives of Quality of Life in Mild Cognitive Impairment and Alzheimer's disease. *Int J Geriatr Psychiatry.* 2004; 19: 256–265

[28] A PubMed literature search did not find other controlled studies of cognition and QoL in dementia.

[29] The Dude, *The Big Lebowski*

[30] Livingston G, et al. Successful ageing in adversity: the LASER–AD longitudinal study. *J Neurol Neurosurg Psychiatry.* 2008;79:641–645. doi:10.1136/jnnp.2007.126706

[Cognitive test] scores were not significantly correlated with either patient- or caregiver-reported QOL scores.[31]

Self-reported QoL was significantly correlated to depression but not to age, dementia severity, behavioural symptoms or memory impairment.... Self-reported QoL did not correlate with the [cognitive test] score.[32]

Quality of life at follow-up correlated significantly with depression and anxiety but not with cognition...Thus, despite deterioration in cognitive abilities and increased dependency, most people with dementia do not view their quality of life as having deteriorated.[33]

QoL and cognitive impairment seem to be relatively independent in mild dementia.[34]

QOL is stable or improves despite the global cognitive deterioration, particularly in the more advanced stages of dementia.[35]

[31] Logsdon RG, et al. Assessing Quality of Life in Older Adults With Cognitive Impairment. *Psychosomatic Medicine*. 2002; 64:510–519

[32] Vogel A, et al. Patient versus informant reported quality of life in the earliest phases of Alzheimer's disease. *Int J Geriatr Psychiatry* 2006; 21: 1132–1138. DOI: 10.1002/gps.1619

[33] Selwood A, et al. Quality of life in dementia—a one-year follow-up study. *Int J Geriatr Psychiatry* 2005; 20: 232–237

[34] Dourado M, et al. Quality of life in mild dementia: patterns of change in self and caregiver ratings over time. *Revista Brasileira de Psiquiatria* 2016;38:294–300. DOI::10.1590/1516-4446-2014-1642

[35] Oudman E, et al. Quality of life in nursing home residents with advanced dementia: a 2-year follow-up. *Psychogeriatrics* 2014; 14: 235–240. DOI: 10.1111/psyg.12062

The lower quality of life previously reported by people with cognitive impairment is due to the greater physical and mental health problems in this population, rather than to cognitive impairment per se.[36]

For many, it may be consoling that QoL is independent of cognitive decline in most people. There are exceptions to this finding, the most obvious being those people who were excluded from studies due to very severe dementia or for behavioral reasons (so-called "neuropsychiatric symptoms" that include delusions, hallucinations, agitation, irritability, and disinhibition, as well as less disruptive symptoms like apathy and depression). It is impossible to know the interior experience of these unfortunate PWD whose difficulties are so affecting and vivid as to inform the fictional depiction of dementia—for instance, Tony Soprano's hallucinating mother, whose demented volatility magnifies the evil of her pre-dementia life, or the aged partner in *Ray Donovan* who is ruled by the bizarre urgings of an inner voice.[37] A survey of neuropsychiatric symptoms in Alzheimer's dementia found that 59%

---

[36] Cooper C, et al. Successful aging in health adversity: results from the National Psychiatric Morbidity Survey. *International Psychogeriatrics* 2009;21(5):861–868. DOI: 10.1017/S104161020900920X

[37] Just as we cannot assume that we are able to judge QoL accurately in people with a more typical dementia course, we cannot not really know that these PWD with hallucinations, delusions, or irritability are indeed suffering. Assessments of neuropsychiatric symptoms in PWD usually rely the Neuropsychiatric Inventory (NPI), a test which relies entirely on proxy reporting. We have already seen how, in mild to moderately severe dementia, proxy reporting is unreliable. Even so, anger, irritability, and apathy are associated with poor QoL in the nondemented, suggesting that their presence may also reduce QoL in the PWD.

had one or no such symptoms, 28% had mood symptoms such as depression or apathy, and 13% had disruptive symptoms like hallucinations and delusions.[38] It is hard to believe that these more extreme and disruptive neuropsychiatric symptoms—delusions, hallucinations, and disinhibition—do not have a negative effect on quality of life. Managing QoL for these PWD is a matter of daily triage, of keeping them safe and easing their unrest. While the medical literature reassures that a demented individual is likely to sustain the same QoL as their undemented peers, the experience of this disturbed minority inspires compassion as well as the hope that it will not happen to oneself.[39]

It is easy to imagine another exception to the finding that QoL is sustained in dementia. Consider how it would feel to be diagnosed with Alzheimer's disease or Mild Cognitive Impairment. You hoped your forgetfulness was normal for age—after all, older people do forget things, correct? But then your physician breaks the bad news. If you are diagnosed with MCI, the diagnosis is typically presented as a stepping-stone to dementia, as if were just a matter of time until dementia develops.[40] This is bad news. You see yourself in a nursing home, alone in an anonymous room, in a wheelchair,

[38] Lyketsos CG, et al. Neuropsychiatric disturbance in Alzheimer's disease clusters into three groups: the Cache County study. *Int J Geriatr Psychiatry* 2001; 16: 1043-1053. DOI: 10.1002/gps.44

[39] Recall that PWD with depression, anxiety, and apathy are included in studies of QoL in dementia, suggesting that presence of these symptoms does not necessarily rule out good QoL.

[40] As we learned in the chapter on Mild Cognitive Impairment, this is a misrepresentation of MCI's actual course, in which about 10% per year convert to AD while the rest either do not progress or revert to normal.

on your legs a blanket spotted with bits of the day's meals and a crossword puzzle provided for "cognitive maintenance," the TV murmuring daytime programming you do not understand, staring at nothing, your diaper wet—in short, the picture of dementia that is the default representation in books and movies. Now, with your new diagnosis and this vivid picture in mind, you are depressed and hopeless, as you should be, for you do not understand that your life will probably be different than the one you picture. Depression in early AD and MCI is not uncommon and accompanies a dip in self-reported QoL, suggesting that reduced QoL in the early stages of dementia may be a reaction to the diagnosis.[41] People with MCI or AD are still adapting to their diagnoses; it is an emotional catch-up period in which the many adaptive techniques noted in this chapter are invoked—age-norming, affirming competencies, using humor, adjusting expectations, shifting goals— but have not yet had their positive effect on QoL. Perhaps the anticipation of disability—like the anticipation of pain—is usually worse than the fact. Planning for the future, particularly if the plans include a spouse or other family, as well as psychologic adaption, may mitigate depression and improve mood and QoL.

There is probably a second cause for the dip and then rise in quality of life in Mild Cognitive Impairment and early Alzheimer's disease: anosognosia. Anosognosia is the lack of awareness of what one does not know. Stated another way, having anosognosia means

[41] Stites SD, et al. Awareness of Mild Cognitive Impairment and Mild Alzheimer's Disease Dementia Diagnoses Associated With Lower Self-Ratings of Quality of Life in Older Adults. *J Gerontol B Psychol Sci Soc Sci* 2017;72(6,):974–985. DOI:10.1093/geronb/gbx100

that one does not know what one does not know.[42] Anosognosia is usually considered an impairment. The math student who is unaware of her lack of understanding of a concept cannot improve her understanding and therefore is likely to miscalculate. Anosognosia is a liability in dementia, too, causing people to underestimate the danger they may pose to themselves in cooking or driving, for example. But anosognosia also has a merciful effect. It may improve QoL.

This makes sense. The person with MCI or the early stages of Alzheimer's disease may be more aware of their cognitive trouble—and hence more depressed—than more progressed cases of AD in which awareness of deficits is lost. One researcher confirms this idea: "Persons with MCI or AD who were aware of their diagnosis reported lower average satisfaction with daily life, basic functioning, and physical wellbeing, and more difficulties in daily life than those who were unaware." Moreover, studies show that as dementia progresses and anosognosia increases, quality of life may also increase: "Overall, patients with severe anosognosia gave higher ratings of QoL, whereas those [with mild or no anosognosia] rated QoL as worse. This shows that a greater awareness of deficits and difficulties (less anosognosia) is related to a poorer perception of QoL, and highlights the relevance of psychological factors in the early stages of the disease (lower [QoL scores are] associated with greater depression and less anosognosia)."[43]

---

[42] Anosognosia is a metacognitive error.

[43] Conde-Sala JL, et al. Clinical Differences in Patients with Alzheimer's Disease According to the Presence or Absence of Anosognosia: Implications for Perceived Quality of Life. *Journal of Alzheimer's Disease* 2013; 33: 1105–1116. DOI 10.3233/JAD-2012-121360

Thus, the decline into severe dementia is, for some, softened by a lack of awareness of the decline. Anosognosia is, in a way, another aspect of the loss of self: in this case, it is the loss of the ability to know oneself. This loss may appear tragic to witnesses—who would be guilty, yet again, of misunderstanding quality of life in dementia.

The best answer to the question, "Is it so bad to be demented?" is "Compared to what?" Compared to mid-life, it is worse to be demented. The unravelling of the mind in dementia does not reveal a leaner mind configured for a special wisdom. In dementia, the mind is diminished, full stop. It is simplified in the worst sense, its "Sequence ravelled out of reach," as Emily Dickinson describes the unstoppable unwinding of the mind in the quotation at the beginning of this book.

But compared to the lives of the non-demented aged, the lives of most people with dementia cannot really be said to be worse. Quality of life tends to decline from middle age onwards whether one is demented or not because healthy middle-aged people inevitably become older people who are increasingly frail, dependent, and have a growing number of medical problems. The demented have their unique difficulties—some people with dementia develop agitation, irritability, hallucinations—and all PWD must adapt, adjusting their expectations for life. But the challenges faced by people with dementia, though different in kind, may not be greater in degree than the challenges faced by the multimorbid aged. Both groups adapt to adversity, and in doing so they maintain value in living. "For most of us," states the quotation at the beginning of this chapter, "it would take a lot more than we think to make us permanently miserable."

As I wrote this chapter, I came across passages in books and movies that made me reflect on the significance for me of the chapter's conclusions. One quotation is from Peter Jackson's movie adaptation of *The Lord of the Rings*. In this scene, orcs have overrun the citadel of Minas Tirith, and Pippin, who is a hobbit and not a fighter, fears death. He looks to Gandalf, a wizard, for courage.

> **Pippin:** I didn't think it would end this way.
>
> **Gandalf:** End? No, the journey doesn't end here. Death is just another path, one that we all must take. The grey rain-curtain of this world rolls back, and all turns to silver glass, and then you see it.
>
> **Pippin:** What, Gandalf? See what?
>
> **Gandalf:** White shores, and beyond, a far green country under a swift sunrise.
>
> **Pippin:** Well, that isn't so bad.
>
> **Gandalf:** No. No, it isn't.

It is tempting to take comfort in Gandalf's words. Loss is figured here not as a separation from normal life but as a kind of arrival at a fresh and hopeful vista. I, too, had hope that my research for this chapter would reveal dementia as both a loss and a gain, as a continuation of the lifelong shaping of the mind, the aged brain but a "grey rain-curtain" behind which a different brain emerges. But such is not the case. Instead, the surprise that life offers is characteristic of what life usually offers: a mix of the good and the bad. Life with dementia is not a matter of the caterpillar becoming a butterfly; it is the much more prosaic effort of the caterpillar learning how to live with its imperfect self, adapting to flightlessness, and adjusting its expectations. A passage from *The Women of Troy*, by Pat Barker, is more to this point. In contrast to Tolkien's description of an arrival, the narrator here describes a departure when, as a boy, he was taken from home to be trained as a priest.

> Once a month, he's allowed to go home, and at first he longs for that day, even marks the days on the ground with a piece of chalky stone, but then increasingly with every visit he ceases to belong in the neighbourhood and even in his own home—as if he were in a fast-moving ship and his mother was just a tiny figure waving from the shore.

When he is first sent away, the boy sees only what he has lost—his mother, his neighborhood, his home. He is desperately homesick, marking the days until the next chance to return. For the boy, it is unthinkable that his love for home could ever change, yet the man looking back at the boy is surprised by how transient was the need for home. Each time the boy returns, and each time he looks back at home from the departing ship, his old life has diminished, until, at last, it has the insignificance of a remote figure on the shore. In adapting to his new life, he gives up the old.

So it is, ideally, in life with dementia. No grey rain-curtain rolls back to reveal a greener world. Instead, as the importance of the old life wanes, we move forward in whatever weather. We are more mindful of what we have than of what we have lost, we seek inspiration, we find the good and overlook the bad, we are thankful for what we enjoy while also looking forward to more, we depend upon on the help of others, and we love the people we love—just as we always have.

🔔 REMEMBER:

✓ For most people, quality of life (QoL) increases from childhood, peaks in middle age, and declines in older age.

✓ QoL usually decreases in old age whether one is demented or not.

✓ Non-demented people are poor at estimating the QoL of people with dementia (PWD).

✓ PWD dementia rate their QoL higher than is expected by people without dementia.

✓ QoL in dementia is not linked to cognitive ability.

✓ Factors that influence QoL in PWD are the same factors that influence QoL in the non-demented

✓ Both the demented and non-demented sustain QoL by adapting to adversity.

✓ QoL in PWD is supported by anosognosia, a dementia-associated lack of awareness of disability.

GENETIC/FAMILIAL FACTORS AND RISK FOR ALZHEIMER'S DISEASE

See footnotes for more information

Background Risk	Age(b)	Gender (c)	Ethnicity (d)	Family History of AD (e)	APOE (g)	APOE +Ethnicity (i)	APOE +Family History (k)	APOE +Family History +African American Ethnicity (l)
10-12% LTR (a)	Age<65: <1%	Female: 20%	Japanese: 6.3%	Anyone: 39%	Any Female E3/E4: (h) 30%	African American E3/E4: 2.3	Any E3/E4: 46.1%	Female E3/E4: 73%
	Age 65-74: 5.3%	Male: 10%	Native American: 10%	Any Female: 43.9%	Any Female E4/E4: (h) 60%	African American E4/E4: 8.75	Any E4/E4: 61.4%	Female E4/E4: 74%
	Age 75-84: 13.8%		Asian and Pacific Islander: 10%	Any Male: 30.9%	Any Male E3/E4: (h) 23%	Chinese any E4: (j) 3.34	Female E3/E4: 50.3%	Male E3/E4: 56%
	Age >85: 34.6%		White: 10%	African American: 57.1 (f)	Any Male E4/E4: (h) 51%	Japanese any E4: (j) 2.39	Female E4/E4: 72.2%	Male E4/E4: 77%
			Hispanic: 14%	White: 43.7% (f)		Hispanic E3/E4: 3.1	Male E3/E4:(m) 38.5%	
			African American: 18%			Hispanic E4/E4: 7.15	Male E4/E4:(m) 35.3%	

a. Lifetime Risk (LTR) to age 80-85

References:

Rajan KB, et al. Population estimate of people with clinical Alzheimer's disease and mild cognitive impairment in the United States (2020–2060). *Alzheimer's Dement.* 2021;1–10. DOI: 10.1002/alz.12362

Goldman JS, et al. Genetic counseling and testing for Alzheimer disease: Joint practice guidelines of the American College of Medical Genetics and the National Society of Genetic Counselors. *Genet Med.* 2011:13(6):597–605. DOI: 10.1097/GIM.0b013e31821d69b8

Bird TD. Genetic Aspects of Alzheimer Disease. *Genet Med.* 2008 April ; 10(4): 231–239. doi:10.1097/GIM.0b013e31816b64dc

Cupples LA, et al. Estimating risk curves for first-degree relatives of patients with Alzheimer's disease: The REVEAL study. *Genet Med.* 2004:6(4):192–196

b. Numbers indicate prevalence of AD in the general population for each age group indicated; not LTR.

Reference:

Rajan KB, et al. Population estimate of people with clinical Alzheimer's disease and mild cognitive impairment in the United States (2020–2060). *Alzheimer's Dement.* 2021;1–10. DOI: 10.1002/alz.12362

c. Numbers indicate Lifetime Risk (LTR). Data from Gender and incidence of dementia in the Framingham Heart Study from mid-adult life. Alz dement, 2015

d. Numbers indicate prevalence of AD in the general population.

References:

Matthews KA, et al. Racial and ethnic estimates of Alzheimer's disease and related dementias in the United States (2015–2060) in adults aged ≥65 years. *Alzheimers Dement.* 2019; 15(1): 17–24. doi:10.1016/j.jalz.2018.06.3063.

Rajan KB, et al. Population estimate of people with clinical Alzheimer's disease and mild cognitive impairment in the United States (2020–2060). *Alzheimer's Dement.* 2021;1–10. DOI: 10.1002/alz.12362

Mehta KM, et al. Systematic review of dementia prevalence and incidence in United States race/ethnic populations. *Alzheimers Dement.* 2017;72-83

e. Lifetime risk. "1ˢᵗ-degree family history" = sibling, child, or parent with Late Onset Alzheimer's Disease (LOAD)

References:

Lautenschlager NT, et al. Risk of dementia among relatives of patients in the MIRAGE study: What is in store for the oldest old? *Neurology.* 1996;46:641-650

Green RC, et al. Risk of Dementia Among White and African American Relatives of Patients With Alzheimer Disease. *JAMA.* 2002;287:329-336

f. Assuming a lifespan of 95 years; LTR is lower in shorter lifespans. For example, the risk for dementia to age 85 among 1ˢᵗ degree relatives of African American patients with AD was 43.7%, while among White participants the risk was 26.9% in Green RC, et al. Risk of Dementia Among White and African American Relatives of Patients With Alzheimer Disease. *JAMA.* 2002;287:329-336.

g. LTR to age 85.

h. Table 3a from Genin E. APOE and Alzheimer disease: a major gene with semi-dominant inheritance. *Molecular Psychiatry.* 2011;16, 903–907. This study does not specify the ethnicities of the participants except that they are from "the west of France and the USA".

See also Slooter AJC, et al. Risk Estimates of Dementia by Apolipoprotein E Genotypes From a Population-Based Incidence Study: The Rotterdam Study. *Arch Neurol.* 1998;55:964-968. In this study, the E4/E3 and E4/4 genotypes were grouped together for a single risk estimate, with the lifetime risk of dementia for any E4 genotype 46% for women and 26% for men.

i. 1) No similar data is available for other ethnicities except Whites, whose risk is assumed to approximate the values in the previous column, "APOE".

2) Numbers in this column are odds ratios or hazard ratios. An OR of 2.0 means that baseline risk is multiplied by two. ORs give an idea of the proportion of increased risk but do not give absolute lifetime risk. Unfortunately, we do not have Lifetime Risk estimates for these ethnic categories.

3) If the literature gives an OR range, then I have presented a median value. For instance, the OR range for African Americans with the E4/E3 genotype is 2.0-2.6, which I report as (2.0+2.6)/2 = 2.3

j. The E4/E3 OR for Chinese is 3.1 and for Japanese it is 4.0. The ORs for Chinese and Japanese with the E4/E4 genotype are unbelievably high—probably due to low sample sizes—and I chose to report only the "any genotype" (E3/4 or E4/4) in the table.

k. 1) APOE genotypes in this case refer not to the genotype of the unaffected family member but to the genotype of the demented 1st degree relative.

2) Numbers are LTR to age 90

3) Reference: Martinez M, et al. Apolipoprotein E e4 Allele and Familial Aggregation of Alzheimer Disease. *Arch Neurol.* 1998;55:810-816

l. 1) Risks for Whites are assumed to approximate the values in the previous column, "APOE+Family History".

2) Numbers are LTR and based on REVEAL studies' data. These are the LTR for AD that genetic counselors showed the participants in the REVEAL study prior to disclosure of

APOE genotype results. The numbers are misleading, calculated as they are using the APOE genotype not of the unaffected 1st degree relatives but on the genotype of the demented relative. I did not find any studies on AD risk in 1st degree
relatives of AD patients that assessed the APOE genotype of
the unaffected relatives of any specified ethnicities.

3) See chapter bibliography for references

m. These data points are counterintuitive. Males with two E4
genes have a lower LTR for AD than males with one E4 gene.

WORKS CITED

Aine CJ, et al. Development and Decline of Memory Functions in Normal, Pathological and Healthy Successful Aging. *Brain Topogr* 2011; 24(3-4): 323–339. DOI: 10.1007/s10548-011-0178-x

Albrecht GL, et al. The disability paradox: high quality of life against all odds. *Social Science & Medicine* 1999;48: 977-988

Allen JS, et al. Normal neuroanatomical variation due to age: The major lobes and a parcellation of the temporal region. *Neurobiology of Aging* 2005;26:1245–1260. DOI: 10.1016/j.neurobiolaging.2005.05.023

Amariglio RE, et al. Specific Subjective Memory Complaints in Older Persons May Indicate Poor Cognitive Function. *J Am Geriatr Soc* 2011;59:1612–1617. DOI: 10.1111/j.1532-5415.2011.03543.x

Artero S, et al. Risk profiles for mild cognitive impairment and progression to dementia are gender specific. *J Neurol Neurosurg Psychiatry* 2008;79(9):979–984. DOI: 10.1136/ jnnp.2007.136903

Arvanitakis Z, et al. Diagnosis and Management of Dementia: Review. *JAMA* 2019;322 (16)

Bang J, et al. Non-Alzheimer's dementia 1: Frontotemporal dementia. *Lancet* 2015;386(10004): 1672–1682. DOI: 10.1016/S0140-6736(15)00461-4

Bertram L, et al. The Genetics of Alzheimer Disease: Back to the Future. *Neuron.* 2010;68. DOI: 10.1016/j.neuron.2010.10.013

Bird TD. Genetic Aspects of Alzheimer Disease. *Genet Med.* 2008;10(4):231–239. DOI: 10.1097/GIM.0b013e31816b64dc

Blacker D, et al. APOE-4 and age at onset of Alzheimer's disease: The NIMH Genetics Initiative. *Neurology.* 1997;48:139-147

Blazer DG, et al. Memory Complaint as a Predictor of Cognitive Decline. A Comparison of African American and White Elders. *Journal of Aging and Health* 1997;9:171-184

Breitner JCS, *et al. APOE*-E4 count predicts age when prevalence of AD increases, then declines: The Cache County Study. *Neurology* 1999;53:321–331

Brickman P, et al. Lottery Winners and Accident Victims: Is Happiness Relative? *Journal of Personality and Social Psychology* 1978;36(8): 917-927

Casey BJ, et al. Imaging the developing brain: what have we learned about cognitive development? *TRENDS in Cognitive Sciences* 2005;9(3)

Chene G, et al. Gender and incidence of dementia in the Framingham Heart Study from mid-adult life. *Alzheimers Dement.* 2015;11(3):310–320. DOI: 10.1016/j.jalz.2013.10.005

Christensen KD, et al. Changes to perceptions of the pros and cons of genetic susceptibility testing after *APOE* genotyping for Alzheimer disease risk. *Genet Med* 2011:13(5):409–414

Christensen KD, et al. Incorporating ethnicity into genetic risk assessment for Alzheimer disease: the REVEAL study experience. *Genet Med.* 2008:10(3):207–214

Clement F, et al. Cognitive complaint in mild cognitive impairment and Alzheimer's disease. *Journal of the International Neuropsychological Society.* 2008;14, 222–232. DOI: 10.10170S1355617708080260

Commissaris CJAM, et al. Subjective forgetfulness in a normal Dutch population: possibilities for health education and other interventions. *Patient Education and Counseling* 1998;34:25–32

Conde-Sala JL, et al. Clinical Differences in Patients with Alzheimer's Disease According to the Presence or Absence of Anosognosia: Implications for Perceived Quality of Life. *Journal of Alzheimer's Disease* 2013; 33: 1105–1116. DOI: 10.3233/JAD-2012-121360

Cooper C, et al. Successful aging in health adversity: results from the National Psychiatric Morbidity Survey. *International Psychogeriatrics* 2009;21(5):861–868. DOI: 10.1017/S104161020900920X

Craik FIM, Bialystok E. Cognition through the lifespan: mechanisms of change. *TRENDS in Cognitive Sciences* 2006;10(3). DOI: 10.1016/j.tics.2006.01.007

Crespo M, et al. Factors associated with quality of life in dementia patients in long-term care. *International Psychogeriatrics* 2013;25:4,577–585. DOI: 10.1017/S1041610212002219

Cupples LA, et al. Estimating risk curves for first-degree relatives of patients with Alzheimer's disease: The REVEAL study. *Genet Med* 2004:6(4):192–196

Cutler DM, et al. Measuring the Health of the U.S. Population. *Brookings Papers on Economic Activity. Microeconomics* 1997, pp. 217-282. https://www.jstor.org/stable/2534757

Demirovic J, et al. Prevalence of Dementia in Three Ethnic Groups: The South Florida Program on Aging and Health. *Ann Epidemiol* 2003;13:472–478

Devi G, et al. Influence of APOE genotype on familial aggregation of AD in an urban population. *Neurology*. 1999;53(4):789-789. DOI: 10.1212/WNL.53.4.789

Dourado M, et al. Quality of life in mild dementia: patterns of change in self and caregiver ratings over time. *Revista Brasileira de Psiquiatria* 2016;38:294–300. DOI: 10.1590/1516-4446-2014-1642

Droess R-M, et al. Quality of life in dementia in perspective. *Dementia* 2006;5(4):533-558. DOI: 10.1177/1471301206069929

El Haj M, et al. "La vie en rose": A positive shift of autobiographical memory in Alzheimer's Disease. *Archives of Gerontology and Geriatrics* 2020; 86:103953. DOI: 10.1016/j.archger.2019.103953

Farrer LA, et al. Apolipoprotein E Genotype in Patients with Alzheimer's Disease: Implications for the Risk of Dementia Among Relatives. *Ann Neurol* 1995;38:797-808

Farrer LA, et al. Effects of age, sex, and ethnicity on the Association Between Apolipoprotein E Genotype and Alzheimer Disease: a Meta-analysis. *JAMA* 1997:278:1349-1356

Gale SA, et al. Dementia. *The American Journal of Medicine* 2018;131:1161–1169. DOI: 10.1016/j.amjmed.2018.01.022

Geda YE, et al. Higher risk of progression to dementia in mild cognitive impairment cases who revert to normal, *Neurology* 2014 (82);317–325

Genin E. APOE and Alzheimer disease: a major gene with semi-dominant inheritance. *Molecular Psychiatry* 2011;16, 903–907

Glodzik-Sobanska L, et al. Subjective Memory Complaints: Presence, Severity and Future Outcome in Normal Older Subjects. *Dement Geriatr Cogn Disord* 2007;24:177–184. DOI: 10.1159/000105604

Goldman JS, et al. Genetic counseling and testing for Alzheimer disease: Joint practice guidelines of the American College of Medical Genetics and the National Society of Genetic

Counselors. *Genet Med.* 2011:13(6):597–605. DOI: 10.1097/GIM.0b013e31821d69b8

Gomperts SN. Lewy Body Dementias: Dementia With Lewy Bodies and Parkinson Disease Dementia. *Continuum* 2016;22(2):435–463

Gooding HC, et al. Genetic susceptibility testing for Alzheimer disease: Motivation to obtain information and control as precursors to coping with increased risk. *Patient Education and Counseling* 2006;64:259–267

Graff-Radford NR, et al. Association Between Apolipoprotein E Genotype and Alzheimer Disease in African American Subjects. *Arch Neurol* 2002;59:594-600

Green RC, et al. Disclosure of *APOE* Genotype for Risk of Alzheimer's Disease. *N Engl J Med* 2009;361:245-54

Green RC, et al. Risk of Dementia Among White and African American Relatives of Patients With Alzheimer Disease. *JAMA* 2002;287:329-336

Growing Old in America: Expectations vs. Reality (Pew Research Center, 2009). https://www.pewresearch.org/social-trends/2009/06/29/growing-old-in-america-expectations-vs-reality/

Gupta S, et al. Rare and Unusual Dementias. *Advances in psychiatric treatment* 2009;15: 364–371 DOI: 10.1192/apt.bp.107.003558

Harada CN, et al. Normal Cognitive Aging. *Clin Geriatr Med* 2013;29(4):737–752. DOI: 10.1016/j.cger.2013.07.002

Havlik RJ, et al. APOE-E4 predicts incident AD in Japanese-American men: The Honolulu–Asia Aging Study. *Neurology* 2000;54:1526–1529

Hebert LE, et al. Age-Specific Incidence of Alzheimer's Disease in a Community Population. *JAMA* 1995;273:1354-1359

Hiraki S, et al. Perceptions of Familial Risk in those Seeking a Genetic Risk Assessment for Alzheimer's Disease. *J Genet Counseling* 2009;18 (2),130-136. DOI: 10.1007/s10897-008-9194-8

Huang W, et al. APOE Genotype, Family History of Dementia, and Alzheimer Disease Risk. A 6-Year Follow-up Study. *Arch Neurol* 2004;61:1930-1934

Jungwirth S, et al. Subjective Memory Complaints and Objective Memory Impairment in the Vienna-Transdanube Aging Community. *JAGS* 2004 52:263–268

Katzman R, et al. Effects of apolipoprotein E on dementia and aging in the Shanghai Survey of Dementia. *Neurology* 1997;49:779-785

King J, et al. Quality of Life in Late-Life Disability: "I Don't Feel Bitter Because I Am in a Wheelchair." *J Am Geriatr Soc* 2012;60:569–576. DOI: 10.1111/j.1532-5415.2011.03844.x

Knight BG, Durbin K. Aging and the effects of emotion on cognition: Implications for psychological interventions for depression and anxiety. *Psych J* 2015;4(1):11–19. DOI:10.1002/pchj.84

Lautenschlager NT, et al. Risk of dementia among relatives of patients in the MIRAGE study: What is in store for the oldest old? *Neurology* 1996;46:641-650

Litvinchuk A, et al. Apolipoprotein E4 reduction with antisense oligonucleotides decreases neurodegeneration in a tauopathy model. *Ann Neurol* 2021;89(5):952-966. DOI: 10.1002/ana.26043

Livingston G, et al. Successful ageing in adversity: the LASER–AD longitudinal study. *J Neurol Neurosurg Psychiatry* 2008;79:641–645. DOI: 10.1136/jnnp.2007.126706

Livingston G, et al. Dementia prevention, intervention, and care: 2020 report of the *Lancet* Commission. *Lancet* 2020;396:413–46. DOI: 10.1016/S0140-6736(20)30367-6

Logsdon RG, et al. Assessing Quality of Life in Older Adults With Cognitive Impairment. *Psychosomatic Medicine* 2002; 64:510–519

Logue MW, et al. A Comprehensive Genetic Association Study of Alzheimer Disease in African Americans. *Arch Neurol* 2011;68(12):1569-1579

Lyketsos CG, et al. A follow-up study of change in quality of life among persons with dementia residing in a long-term care facility. *Int J Geriatr Psychiatry* 2003;18:275–281

Lyketsos CG, et al. Neuropsychiatric disturbance in Alzheimer's disease clusters into three groups: the Cache County study. *Int J Geriatr Psychiatry* 2001;16:1043-1053. DOI: 10.1002/gps.44

Maestre G, et al. Apolipoprotein E and Alzheimer's Disease: Ethnic Variation in Genotypic Risks. *Ann Neurol* 1995;37:254-259

Mahley R. Apolipoprotein E: from cardiovascular disease to neurodegenerative disorders. *J Mol Med* 2016; 94:739–746. DOI: 10.1007/s00109-016-1427-y

Makovski TT, et al. Multimorbidity and quality of life: Systematic literature review and meta- analysis. *Ageing Research Reviews* 2019;53:100903. DOI: 10.1016/j.arr.2019.04.005

Manly JJ. Frequency and course of mild cognitive impairment in a multiethnic community. *Ann Neurology* 2008;63 (4):494–506. DOI: 10.1002/ana.21326

Marek S, et al. Reproducible brain-wide association studies require thousands of individuals. *Nature* online, March 2022

Marengoni A, et al. Aging with multimorbidity: A systematic review of the literature. *Ageing Research Reviews* 2010;10:430–439

Martinez M, et al. Apolipoprotein E e4 Allele and Familial Aggregation of Alzheimer Disease. *Arch Neurol* 1998;55:810-816

Matthews KA, et al. Racial and ethnic estimates of Alzheimer's disease and related dementias in the United States (2015–2060) in adults aged ≥65 years. *Alzheimers Dement* 2019; 15(1): 17–24. DOI: 10.1016/j.jalz.2018.06.3063

Mehta KM, et al. Systematic review of dementia prevalence and incidence in United States race/ethnic populations. *Alzheimers Dement* 2017;72-83

Melgarejo JD, et al. Nighttime Blood Pressure Interacts with *APOE* Genotype to Increase the Risk of Incident Dementia of the Alzheimer's Type in Hispanics. *J Alzheimers Dis* 2020; 77(2): 569–579. DOI: 10.3233/JAD-200430

Mitchell AJ, Shiri-Feshki A. Rate of progression of mild cognitive impairment to dementia—meta-analysis of 41 robust inception cohort studies. *Acta Psychiatr Scand* 2009;119(4):252–65

Mozley CG, et al. 'Not knowing where I am doesn't mean I don't know what I like: cognitive impairment and quality of life responses in elderly people. *Int J Geriat Psychiatry* 1999;14:776-783

Murrell JR, et al. Association of Apolipoprotein E Genotype and Alzheimer Disease in African Americans. *Arch Neurol* 2006 March ; 63(3): 431–434. DOI: 10.1001/archneur.63.3.431

Myers RH. Apolipoprotein E €4 association with dementia in a population-based study: The Framingham Study. *Neurology* 1996;46:673-677

Netuveli G, et al. Quality of life in older ages. *British Medical Bulletin* 2008;85:113–126. DOI: 10.1093/bmb/ldn003

Oudman E, et al. Quality of life in nursing home residents with advanced dementia: a 2-year follow-up. *Psychogeriatrics* 2014;14:235–240. DOI: 10.1111/psyg.12062

Pandya SY, et al. Does mild cognitive impairment always lead to dementia? A review. *Journal of the Neurological Sciences* 2016;369:57–62. DOI: 10.1016/j.jns.2016.07.055

Paradise MB, et al. Subjective memory complaints, vascular risk factors and psychological distress in the middle-aged: a cross-sectional study. *BMC Psychiatry* 2011;11:108

Park DC, et al. Models of Visuospatial and Verbal Memory Across the Adult Life Span. *Psychology and Aging* 2002;17 (2): 299–320. DOI: 10.1037//0882-7974.17.2.299

Park DC, Reuter-Lorenz P. The Adaptive Brain: Aging and Neurocognitive Scaffolding. *Annu Rev Psychol* 2009;60: 173–196. DOI: 10.1146/annurev.psych.59.103006.093656

Paul Slovic, et al. *Facts and Fears: Societal Perception of Risk*, in NA - Advances in Consumer Research Volume 08, eds. Kent B. Monroe, Ann Abor, MI. 1981

Payami H, et al. Prospective Study of Cognitive Health in the Elderly (Oregon Brain Aging Study): Effects of Family History and Apolipoprotein E Genotype. *Am J Hum Genet* 1997;60:948-956

Perrotin A, et al. Metamemory monitoring in mild cognitive impairment: Evidence of a less accurate episodic feeling-of-knowing. *Neuropsychologia* 2007;45:2811–2826. DOI: 10.1016/j.neuropsychologia.2007.05.003

Peterson R. Mild Cognitive Impairment. *N Engl J Med* 2011;364:2227-34

Qin Z, et al. Longitudinal Comparison of Stability and Sensitivity in Quality of Life Scores Among Nursing Home Residents With and Without Diagnoses of Alzheimer's Disease and Related Dementias. *Innovation in Aging* 2021;5(3):1–11. DOI: 10.1093/geroni/igab024

Qui C, et al. Risk and protective effects of the APOE gene towards Alzheimer's disease in the Kungsholmen project: variation by age and sex. *J Neurol Neurosurg Psychiatry* 2004;75:828–833. DOI: 10.1136/jnnp.2003.021493

Rajan KB, et al. Population estimate of people with clinical Alzheimer's disease and mild cognitive impairment in the United States (2020–2060). *Alzheimer's Dement* 2021;1–10. DOI: 10.1002/alz.12362

Ravaglia G, et al. Mild cognitive impairment: epidemiology and dementia risk in an elderly Italian population. *J Am Geriatr Soc* 2008;56 (1): 51–58. DOI: 10.1111/j.1532-5415.2007.01503.x

Ready RE, et al. Patient versus informant perspectives of Quality of Life in Mild Cognitive Impairment and Alzheimer's disease. *Int J Geriatr Psychiatry* 2004; 19: 256–265

Reduced apolipoprotein €4 allele frequency in the oldest old Alzheimer's patients and cognitively normal individuals. *Neurology* 1994;44:1513-1516

Richard Easterlin. Life cycle happiness and its sources Intersections of psychology, economics, and demography. *Journal of Economic Psychology* 2006;27:463–482. DOI: 10.1016/j.joep.2006.05.002

Riis J, et al. Ignorance of Hedonic Adaptation to Hemodialysis: A Study Using Ecological Momentary Assessment. *Journal of Experimental Psychology: General* 2005;134(1):3–9. DOI: 10.1037/0096-3445.134.1.3

Rippon GA, et al. Familial Alzheimer Disease in Latinos: Interaction Between APOE, Stroke and Estrogen Replacement. *Neurology* 2006; 66(1): 35–40. DOI: 10.1212/01.wnl.0000191300.38571.3e

Roberts JS, et al. Reasons for Seeking Genetic Susceptibility Testing Among First-Degree Relatives of People With Alzheimer Disease. *Alzheimer Disease and Associated Disorders* 2003;17(2):86–93

Roberts RO, et al. Higher risk of progression to dementia in mild cognitive impairment cases who revert to normal, *Neurology* 2014;82:317–325

Sachdev PS, et al. Factors predicting reversion from mild cognitive impairment to normal cognitive functioning: a population-based study. *PLoS One* 2013;8(3):1–10

Sanford A. Mild Cognitive Impairment. *Clin Geriatr Med* 2017;33:25–337. DOI: 10.1016/j.cger.2017.02.005

Schmidtke K, et al. The Syndrome of Functional Memory Disorder: Definition, Etiology, and Natural Course. *Am J Geriatr Psychiatry* 2008;16:981–988

Schu MC, et al. "The Genetics of Alzheimer's Disease". From: Hampel H, Carrillo MC (eds): Alzheimer's Disease – Modernizing Concept, Biological Diagnosis and Therapy. *Adv Biol Psychiatry* 2012;28:15–29

Selwood A, et al. Quality of life in dementia—a one-year follow-up study. *Int J Geriatr Psychiatry* 2005; 20: 232–237

Singer T, et al. The Fate of Cognition in Very Old Age: Six-Year Longitudinal Findings in the Berlin Aging Study (BASE). *Psychology and Aging* 2003;18(2):18–331. DOI: 10.1037/0882-7974.18.2.318

Slooter AJC, et al. Risk Estimates of Dementia by Apolipoprotein E Genotypes From a Population-Based Incidence Study: The Rotterdam Study. *Arch Neurol* 1998;55:964-968

Snitz, BE, et al. Subjective memory complaints and concurrent memory performance in older patients of primary care providers. *J Int Neuropsychol Soc* 2008;14(6):1004–1013. DOI: 10.1017/S1355617708081332

Staffaroni AM, et al. Neuroimaging in dementia. *Semin Neurol* 2017;37(5): 510–537. DOI: 10.1055/s-0037-1608808

Steeman E, et al. Living with dementia from the perspective of older people: Is it a positive story? *Aging & Mental Health* 2007;11:2, 119-130. DOI: 10.1080/13607860600963364

Steffi G, et al. Do memory complaints indicate the presence of cognitive impairment? – Results of a field study. *Eur Arch Psychiatry Clin Neurosci* 1999;249:97–204

Stites SD, et al. Awareness of Mild Cognitive Impairment and Mild Alzheimer's Disease Dementia Diagnoses Associated With Lower Self-Ratings of Quality of Life in Older Adults. *J Gerontol B Psychol Sci Soc Sci* 2017;72(6,):974–985. DOI: 10.1093/geronb/gbx100

Stone AA, et al. A snapshot of the age distribution of psychological well-being in the United States. *PNAS* 2010;107(22):9985–9990

Sweeting H, et al. Dementia and the phenomenon of social death. *Sociology of Health & Illness* 1997;19(1):93-117

Tang M-X, et al. Incidence of AD in African-Americans, Caribbean Hispanics, and Caucasians in northern Manhattan. *Neurology* 2001;56:49–56

Tang M-X, et al. Relative Risk of Alzheimer Disease and Age-at-Onset Distributions, Based on APOE Genotypes among Elderly African Americans, Caucasians, and Hispanics in New York City. *Am J Hum Genet* 1996;58:574-584

Tang M-X, et al. The APOE-e4 Allele and the Risk for Alzheimer's Disease Among African Americans, Whites, and Hispanics. *JAMA* 1998;279:751-755

Van der Zon A, et al. Two-Year Course of Quality of Life in Nursing Home Residents with Dementia. *Am J Geriatr Psychiatry* 2018; 26:754–764. DOI: 10.1016/j.jagp.2018.01.202

Vogel A, et al. Patient versus informant reported quality of life in the earliest phases of Alzheimer's disease. *Int J Geriatr Psychiatry* 2006; 21: 1132–1138. DOI: 10.1002/gps.1619

Williams MA, Malm J. Diagnosis and Treatment of Idiopathic Normal Pressure Hydrocephalus. *Continuum* 2016;22(2):579-599

Wim Groot. Adaptation and scale of reference bias in self-assessments of quality of life. *Journal of Health Economics* 2000;19:403–420. DOI: 10.1016/S0167-6296(99)00037-5

Woods RT, et al. What contributes to a good quality of life in early dementia? awareness and the QoL-AD: a cross-sectional study. *Health and Quality of Life Outcomes* 2014;12:94

Yoshizawa T, et al. Dose-dependent Association of Apolipoprotein E Allele €4 with Late-Onset, Sporadic Alzheimer's Disease. *Ann Neurol* 1994;36:656-657

Zaninotto P, et al. Age trajectories of quality of life among older adults: results from the English Longitudinal Study of Ageing. *Qual Life Res* 2009;18:1301–1309. DOI 10.1007/s11136-009-9543-6

Zick CD, et al. Genetic Testing For Alzheimer's Disease And Its Impact On Insurance Purchasing Behavior. *Health Affairs* 2005;24(2):483-490. DOI: 10.1377/hlthaff.24.2.483

2021 Alzheimer's Disease Facts and Figures. *Alzheimers Dement* 2021;17(3)

2022 Alzheimer's disease facts and figures. *Alzheimers Dement* 2022;18(4):700-789

Made in United States
North Haven, CT
02 May 2024

52035927R00124